HEALTH LITERACY, eHEALTH, and COMMUNICATION

PUTTING THE CONSUMER FIRST

WORKSHOP SUMMARY

Lyla M. Hernandez, *Rapporteur*

Roundtable on Health Literacy

Board on Population Health and Public Health Practice

INSTITUTE OF MEDICINE
OF THE NATIONAL ACADEMIES

THE NATIONAL ACADEMIES PRESS
Washington, D.C.
www.nap.edu

THE NATIONAL ACADEMIES PRESS   500 Fifth Street, N.W.   Washington, DC 20001

NOTICE: The project that is the subject of this report was approved by the Governing Board of the National Research Council, whose members are drawn from the councils of the National Academy of Sciences, the National Academy of Engineering, and the Institute of Medicine.

This project was supported by contracts between the National Academy of Sciences and the Academy for Educational Development (Unnumbered Award); Affinity Health Plan (Unnumbered Award), Kaiser Permanente (Unnumbered Award); American Academy of Family Physicians (Unnumbered Award); Merck & Co., Inc. (Unnumbered Award); Pfizer Institute (Unnumbered Award); Department of Health and Human Services (N01-OD-4-2139, TO#148); GlaxoSmithKline (G050002912). Any opinions, findings, conclusions, or recommendations expressed in this publication are those of the author(s) and do not necessarily reflect the view of the organizations or agencies that provided support for this project.

International Standard Book Number-13:   978-0-309-12642-7
International Standard Book Number-10:   0-309-12642-8

Additional copies of this report are available from the National Academies Press, 500 Fifth Street, N.W., Lockbox 285, Washington, DC 20055; (800) 624-6242 or (202) 334-3313 (in the Washington metropolitan area); Internet, http://www.nap.edu.

For more information about the Institute of Medicine, visit the IOM home page at: **www.iom.edu.**

Copyright 2009 by the National Academy of Sciences. All rights reserved.

Printed in the United States of America

The serpent has been a symbol of long life, healing, and knowledge among almost all cultures and religions since the beginning of recorded history. The serpent adopted as a logotype by the Institute of Medicine is a relief carving from ancient Greece, now held by the Staatliche Museen in Berlin.

Suggested citation: IOM (Institute of Medicine). 2009. *Health Literacy, eHealth, and Communication: Putting the Consumer First: Workshop Summary.* Washington, DC: The National Academies Press.

*"Knowing is not enough; we must apply.
Willing is not enough; we must do."*
—Goethe

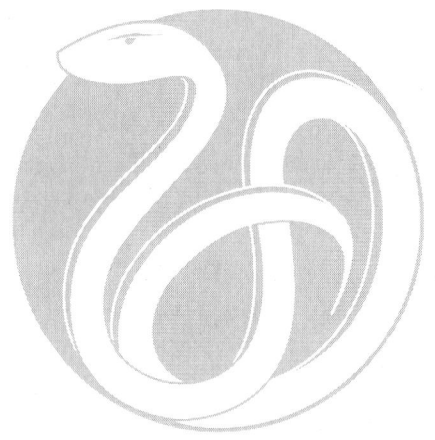

INSTITUTE OF MEDICINE
OF THE NATIONAL ACADEMIES

Advising the Nation. Improving Health.

THE NATIONAL ACADEMIES
Advisers to the Nation on Science, Engineering, and Medicine

The **National Academy of Sciences** is a private, nonprofit, self-perpetuating society of distinguished scholars engaged in scientific and engineering research, dedicated to the furtherance of science and technology and to their use for the general welfare. Upon the authority of the charter granted to it by the Congress in 1863, the Academy has a mandate that requires it to advise the federal government on scientific and technical matters. Dr. Ralph J. Cicerone is president of the National Academy of Sciences.

The **National Academy of Engineering** was established in 1964, under the charter of the National Academy of Sciences, as a parallel organization of outstanding engineers. It is autonomous in its administration and in the selection of its members, sharing with the National Academy of Sciences the responsibility for advising the federal government. The National Academy of Engineering also sponsors engineering programs aimed at meeting national needs, encourages education and research, and recognizes the superior achievements of engineers. Dr. Charles M. Vest is president of the National Academy of Engineering.

The **Institute of Medicine** was established in 1970 by the National Academy of Sciences to secure the services of eminent members of appropriate professions in the examination of policy matters pertaining to the health of the public. The Institute acts under the responsibility given to the National Academy of Sciences by its congressional charter to be an adviser to the federal government and, upon its own initiative, to identify issues of medical care, research, and education. Dr. Harvey V. Fineberg is president of the Institute of Medicine.

The **National Research Council** was organized by the National Academy of Sciences in 1916 to associate the broad community of science and technology with the Academy's purposes of furthering knowledge and advising the federal government. Functioning in accordance with general policies determined by the Academy, the Council has become the principal operating agency of both the National Academy of Sciences and the National Academy of Engineering in providing services to the government, the public, and the scientific and engineering communities. The Council is administered jointly by both Academies and the Institute of Medicine. Dr. Ralph J. Cicerone and Dr. Charles M. Vest are chair and vice chair, respectively, of the National Research Council.

www.national-academies.org

MEMBERS OF THE PLANNING GROUP FOR THE WORKSHOP ON HEALTH LITERACY, eHEALTH, AND COMMUNICATION: PUTTING THE CONSUMER FIRST

CAROLYN COCOTAS, Director, Affinity Health Plan
ARTHUR CULBERT, Senior Advisor to the Missouri Foundation for Health
JANET M. MARCHIBRODA, Chief Executive Officer of the eHealth Initiative and the eHealth Foundation
RUTH PARKER, Associate Professor of Medicine, Emory University School of Medicine
YOLANDA PARTIDA, Director, National Program Office, University of California, San Francisco, Fresno Center for Medical Education and Research
JOSHUA SEIDMAN, President, Center for Information Therapy

IOM planning committees are solely responsible for organizing the workshop, identifying topics, and choosing speakers. The responsibility for the published workshop summary rests with the workshop rapporteur and the institution.

ROUNDTABLE ON HEALTH LITERACY

GEORGE ISHAM (*Chair*), Medical Director and Chief Health Officer, HealthPartners
SHARON E. BARRETT, Association of Clinicians for the Underserved
CAROLYN COCOTAS, Director, Affinity Health Plan
MICHAEL L. DAVIS, Vice President, General Mills
BARBARA A. DEBUONO, Senior Medical Director/Group Leader, Pfizer, Inc.
DEBBIE FRITZ, Director, GlaxoSmithKline
LINDA HARRIS, Acting Team Leader, Health Communication and eHealth Team, U.S. Department of Health and Human Services
BETSY L. HUMPHREYS, Deputy Director, National Institutes of Health
LINDA JOHNSTON-LLOYD, Senior Advisor, Health Resources and Services Administration, Center for Quality
JEAN KRAUSE, Executive Vice President and CEO, American College of Physicians Foundation
DENNIS MILNE, Vice President, Patient Education, American Heart Association
RUTH PARKER, Emory University School of Medicine
YOLANDA PARTIDA, Director, National Program Office, University of California, San Francisco, Fresno Center for Medical Education & Research
KYU BAK LOUIS RHEE, Director, Office of Innovation and Program Coordination, National Center on Minority and Health Disparities, National Institutes of Health
ZORI RODRIGUEZ, Health Disparities Manager, American Academy of Family Physicians
WILLIAM SMITH, Academy for Educational Development
CAROL TEUTSCH, Director, Medical Services, Merck & Co.
WINSTON F. WONG, Clinical Director, Community Benefit, Kaiser Permanente
SABRA WOOLLEY, National Cancer Institute
ANTRONETTE YANCEY, Associate Professor of Health Services and Director, Doctorate in Public Health Program, University of California, School of Public Health

---

IOM forums and roundtables do not issue, review, or approve individual documents. The responsibility for the published workshop summary rests with the workshop rapporteur and the institution.

Study Staff

LYLA M. HERNANDEZ, Staff Director, Roundtable on Health Literacy
KRISTINA SHULKIN, Senior Project Assistant (until July 2008)
ERIN RUSCH, Senior Project Assistant (from August 2008)
ROSE MARIE MARTINEZ, Director, Board on Population Health and
   Public Health Practice
HOPE R. HARE, Administrative Assistant

Reviewers

This report has been reviewed in draft form by persons chosen for their diverse perspectives and technical expertise, in accordance with procedures approved by the National Research Council's Report Review Committee. The purpose of this independent review is to provide candid and critical comments that will assist the institution in making its published report as sound as possible and to ensure that the report meets institutional standards for objectivity, evidence, and responsiveness to the study charge. The review comments and draft manuscript remain confidential to protect the integrity of the deliberative process. We wish to thank the following individuals for their review of this report:

Don E. Detmer, American Medical Informatics Association
Jessie Gruman, Center for the Advancement of Health
Ida Sim, Center for Clinical and Translational Informatics, University of California, San Francisco School of Medicine
Maria E. White, Office of Equal Opportunity and Civil Rights, Health Resources and Services Administration, U.S. Department of Health and Human Services

Although the reviewers listed above have provided many constructive comments and suggestions, they were not asked to endorse the conclusions or recommendations, nor did they see the final draft of the report before its release. The review of this report was overseen by **Hugh Tilson**, Public Health Leadership Program, University of North Carolina School of Public Health. Appointed by the Institute of Medicine, he was responsible for making certain that an independent examination of this report was carried out in accordance with institutional procedures and that all review comments were carefully considered. Responsibility for the final content of this report rests entirely with the author and the institution.

Acknowledgments

Without the support of the sponsors of the Institute of Medicine Roundtable on Health Literacy, it would not have been possible to plan and conduct the workshop, Health Literacy, eHealth, and Communication, which this report summarizes. Sponsors from the Department of Health and Human Services are the Health Resources and Services Administration, the Office of Disease Prevention and Health Promotion, and the National Cancer Institute. Non-federal sponsorship was provided by the Academy for Education Development, Affinity Health Plan, the American Academy of Family Physicians Foundation, GlaxoSmithKline, Kaiser Permanente, Merck & Co., Inc., and Pfizer, Inc.

The Roundtable wishes to express its gratitude to the expert speakers whose presentations provided an overview of eHealth and communication challenges as well as describing consumer-oriented eHealth systems and guides for developing successful health information technology. These speakers were Cindy Brach, Dawn Gauthier, Rita Kukafka, Janet Marchibroda, Kim Nazi, Cameron D. Norman, Anthony Rodgers, Joshua Seidman, and Cynthia Solomon. Thanks also go to Charles Friedman and Linda Harris for their presentations on health literacy, health information technology, and Healthy People 2020.

The Roundtable wishes to thank the planning committee members for their work in putting together an excellent workshop agenda. Members of the planning committee were Carolyn Cocotas, Arthur Culbert, Janet Marchibroda, Ruth Parker, Yolanda Partida, and Joshua Seidman. Thanks also go to George Isham for moderating the entire workshop.

Contents

1 INTRODUCTION 1

2 OVERVIEW OF ISSUES 3
Overview of eHealth, 3
Skills Essential for eHealth, 10
Strategies for Raising Health Literacy in Arizona Medicaid
  Members: New Approaches for State Medicaid "Health
  Knowledge Builders," 15
Discussion, 21

3 OUTCOMES AND CHALLENGES OF eHEALTH APPROACHES:
  PANEL 1 29
Internet Approaches for eHealth in Low-Literacy and Limited-
  English-Proficiency Populations, 29
My Health*e*Vet, 36
Discussion, 40

4 OUTCOMES AND CHALLENGES OF eHEALTH APPROACHES:
  PANEL 2 47
Using Technology to Improve Migrant Health Care Delivery, 47
A User-Centered Personal Health Record: The Design and
  Development of the Shared Care Plan, 54
Observations from the Exam Room: Patient-Centered HIT
  Implementation in Diverse Practice Settings, 63
Discussion, 67

5	EMERGING TOOLS AND STRATEGIES	73

A Guide for Developing and Purchasing Successful Health Information Technology, 73
Discussion, 77
Health Literacy, Health Information Technology, and Healthy People 2020, 78
Discussion, 80

6	CONCLUDING DISCUSSION	85

REFERENCES	89

APPENDIXES

A	GLOSSARY OF TERMS	95
B	WORKSHOP AGENDA	101
C	WORKSHOP SPEAKER BIOSKETCHES	105

TABLES

2-1 Seven-Stage Framework for Assessing and Tracking the Development of Health Information Exchange Initiatives at the State and Local Levels, 8
2-2 Snapshot of Web Utilization Trends/Data January 2008 to February 2008, 19

3-1 Health Information Seeking by Current Internet Use, 31
3-2 Comparison of Principles of Web 2.0 and Web 1.0, 34

FIGURES

2-1 eHealth infrastructure of Medicaid system transformation, 17

3-1 Trust in sources of health information, 32

4-1 Patient dashboard, 49
4-2 Task, 58
4-3 Care team members, 60
4-4 Add diagnosis, 60

5-1 Simple design, 75

1

Introduction

Many observers believe that the use of emerging interactive health information technologies, often referred to as eHealth,[1] can help to improve the quality, capacity, and efficiency of the health care system. eHealth has the potential to improve access to the health care system for traditionally underserved populations and to increase the capacity to provide tailoring and customization for individual patients and consumers (Ahern et al., 2006). eHealth systems can also improve clinical decision making and adherence to clinical guidelines; provide reminder systems for patients and clinicians, thereby improving compliance with preventive service protocols; provide more immediate access to laboratory and radiology results; and, when integrated with clinical decision support systems, help to prevent many errors and adverse events (IOM, 2003).

While eHealth has many potential benefits, some observers have expressed concern that these systems could increase health care disparities by helping mainly those individuals and communities with greater resources. Recent reports show that health care disparities do exist between advantaged and underserved populations (IOM, 2002). Underserved populations generally include ethnic minorities, people in lower

---

[1] It should be noted that throughout the report, speakers use different definitions of the term eHealth in their presentations. This is not surprising since there is no agreed upon definition for the term. In fact, Oh and colleagues (2005) found 51 different definitions for the term eHealth. Since a workshop summary must accurately represent the concepts and ideas of each speaker, no attempt can be made to ensure consistency of definitions across presentations.

socioeconomic groups, and people with lower educational and reading levels. These populations also tend to have limited access to computer technology (Eng et al., 1998).

Furthermore, even if it were possible to ensure equal access to technology, some user groups find it extremely difficult to take advantage of such technology. The average U.S. adult reads on just an eighth-grade level, for example, while most websites are designed for people whose reading level is much higher (Berland et al., 2001). In particular it is the elderly and those with limited literacy and number skills who are most likely to have low health literacy and thus be least able to take advantage of new health technologies.

The Institute of Medicine Roundtable on Health Literacy serves to educate the public, press, and policy makers regarding issues of health literacy. Given the importance of health literacy issues in eHealth, the Roundtable decided to hold a workshop to explore and discuss strategies for improving the ways in which information and communication technologies address the needs of those with low health literacy and language barriers. A planning group designed a workshop to answer the following questions:

- What is the current status of communications technology, particularly electronic records systems?
- What are the challenges of communication technology used for populations with low health literacy?
- What are the strategies for increasing the benefit of these technologies for populations with low health literacy?

The workshop was moderated by George Isham. As the presentations in this workshop demonstrate, tremendous resources are being directed toward the development of health information technologies. While the vast majority of these resources are being devoted to systems that focus on physicians and health institutions, some notable efforts, such as those presented in this workshop, have been made to extend the use of these new technologies to patients. The first panel provided an overview of the issues, including a broad examination of eHealth, skills essential for eHealth, and a discussion of communication inequalities. The next two panels used specific examples to explore the challenges and outcomes of different strategies for addressing health literacy issues in eHealth. The final panel discussed the use of emerging tools in developing eHealth systems. The following workshop summary is organized according to the panel presentations.

2

Overview of Issues

OVERVIEW OF eHEALTH

Janet M. Marchibroda, M.B.A.
Chief Executive Officer, eHealth Initiative and eHealth Foundation

Implementation of eHealth[1] and health information technologies is seen by many observers as an effective way to address current concerns about the quality and safety of the U.S. health care system. Among those concerns are the facts that U.S. adults receive only about half of recommended health care services (McGlynn et al., 2003), that less than 50 percent of adults receive the preventive and screening tests called for in guidelines for their age and sex (Commonwealth Fund, 2006), that preventable medical errors in hospitals result in around 100,000 deaths per year (IOM, 2000), and that there are 1.5 million preventable adverse drug events each year (IOM, 2007).

The rising costs of health care are another major concern that eHealth may help address. By 2016, health care spending in the United States is expected to increase from the current 16 percent of the gross domestic

---

[1] There is an ongoing project devoted to determining definitions of various concepts in eHealth and information technology, however, for purposes of this presentation the following definition applies. *eHealth* "involves simplifying and handling processes relating to information, communication and transactions within and between health care institutions and professionals by utilizing information and telecommunications technologies." (Deutsche Telekom, 2008).

product to 20 percent or $4 trillion (American Academy of Orthopedic Surgeons, 2007). Health insurance premiums for workers and their employees have increased by 78 percent since 2000, while workers' earnings have risen by only 19 percent over the same time period (Kaiser Family Foundation and Health Research and Educational Trust, 2006). Twenty-one percent of employers report it is "very likely" that they will increase the amount that employees pay for health insurance in the coming year, while another 28 percent report it "somewhat likely" that they will do so (Kaiser Family Foundation, 2006).

In the year 2000, 12.7 percent of the U.S. population was age 65 or older. That number is expected to grow to 20 percent by the year 2030 (U.S. Bureau of the Census, 2000), a factor that will contribute to the challenges facing the health care system as it strives to address chronic conditions of the population. In 2000 more than 125 million people in the United States had at least one chronic care condition, and it is predicted that the number will reach 157 million by 2020 (Wu and Green, 2000). Seventy-eight percent of all health care spending in 1998 was focused on those with chronic conditions (Partnership for Solutions, 2004). Himmelstein and colleagues (2005) estimate that medical issues are a major cause of bankruptcy in the United States. Furthermore, there are key challenges concerning access to care and the problems of the 47 million uninsured Americans, problems which many states are now trying to address through health care reform.

The health care debate that will take place over the coming years will likely include all of these issues. And while health care policymakers are focusing on these issues, consumers are also weighing in. A survey by the Kaiser Family Foundation found that more than half of all those surveyed were dissatisfied with the quality of health care and that almost one-third of those indicated they were "very dissatisfied." In addition, 81 percent of those surveyed were dissatisfied with the cost of health care in the United States, with more than 50 percent of the respondents describing themselves as being very dissatisfied (Kaiser Family Foundation and Health Research and Educational Trust, 2006).

When a recent survey by The Commonwealth Fund asked health care opinion leaders to rate the effectiveness of several key strategies for improving the quality and safety of health care, the highest-rated strategy was to accelerate the development and deployment of health information technology. In particular, 67 percent of respondents thought that accelerating adoption of health information technologies would be an effective or highly effective strategy for improving health care, compared with 59 percent for public reporting of provider performance on quality measures, 51 percent for financial incentives for improved quality of care, 50 percent for stronger regulatory oversight of providers, and 39 percent for national voluntary quality campaigns (Shea et al., 2007).

A variety of data support health information technology (IT) as an effective approach to improve quality, safety, and efficiency. For example, the Center for Information Technology Leadership (CITL) in Boston issued a series of reports examining the value and role of health IT. One study indicated that 100 percent adoption of Computerized Provider Order Entry (CPOE) in the ambulatory care environment could save $44 billion annually in reduced medication, radiology, laboratory, and hospitalization expenditures (Johnston et al., 2003). That same study found that use of IT could prevent more than a million adverse drug events and 190,000 hospitalizations per year. A more recent study from CITL indicates standardized health care information exchange could, if fully implemented, result in annual savings of $86.8 billion. This would also mean direct financial benefits for providers and other stakeholders (Walker et al., 2005).

Additional data support the importance of IT as a strategy for addressing various challenges of the health care system. Research conducted at the Brigham and Women's Hospital in Boston concluded that the use of CPOE cut error rates by 55 percent, from 10.7 to 4.9 per 1,000 patient days (Bates et al., 1998). A Kaiser Permanente study of intensive-care patients found that the use of a CPOE system resulted in a 75 percent decrease in incidents of allergic drug reactions and excessive drug dosages. There was also a decrease in the average time spent in the intensive care unit from 4.9 days to 2.7 days. These reductions led to a 25 percent cost savings (Raymond and Dold, 2002).

How, then, should the health care industry move forward with information technology in order to address its various challenges? In 2007, working from a poll of more than 200 organizations across every sector of health care, the eHealth Initiative[2] developed a blueprint that provides a common vision for shared action. The purpose of the blueprint is to provide some initial ideas about how to move forward with the implementation of eHealth and information technology as a way of improving health care. Much of the plan is based on work by Ed Wagner who put

---

[2] "The eHealth Initiative and the Foundation for eHealth Initiative are independent, non-profit affiliated organizations whose missions are the same: to drive improvement in the quality, safety, and efficiency of healthcare through information and information technology. Both organizations are focused on engaging multiple and diverse stakeholders—including hospitals and other healthcare organizations, clinician groups, consumer and patient groups, employers and purchasers, health plans, healthcare information technology organizations, manufacturers, public health agencies, academic and research institutions, and public sector stakeholders—to define and then implement specific actions that will address the quality, safety and efficiency challenges of our healthcare system through the use of interoperable information technology" (eHealth Initiative and Foundation for eHealth Initiative, 2008a).

forward the chronic care model[3] and talked about ways to drive health care improvement, laying out a number of strategies, such as engaging consumers, transforming care delivery, and improving population health. Wagner also examined how eHealth and health information technology can support those key health care improvement strategies. In addition to its ideas for moving forward with eHealth, the blueprint also discusses approaches to aligning incentives and addresses important issues in privacy and confidentiality. The shared vision of the eHealth Initiative blueprint describes a high-performing health care system as one in which

- all those engaged in the care of the patient are linked together in secure and interoperable environments; and
- the decentralized flow of clinical health information directly enables the most comprehensive, patient-centered, safe, efficient, effective, timely and equitable delivery of care where and when it is needed most—at the point of care (Marchibroda, 2008).

Components of eHealth include electronic health records (EHRs)[4] and personal health records[5] (PHRs). There are also a number of new consumer-facing applications, some of which are not referred to as PHRs but which serve a similar purpose as they provide patients with access to their own health information as they move among providers and health plans. Health information exchange is another major component of eHealth. This refers to the electronic exchange of data across organiza-

---

[3] The Chronic Care Model was developed by Ed Wagner, M.D., M.P.H., director of the MacColl Institute for Healthcare Innovation, Group Health Cooperative of Puget Sound and colleagues of the Improving Chronic Illness program with support from the Robert Wood Johnson Foundation.

[4] An EHR system includes "(1) longitudinal collection of electronic health information for and about persons, where health information is defined as information pertaining to the health of an individual or health care provided to an individual; (2) immediate electronic access to person- and population-level information by authorized, and only authorized, users; (3) provision of knowledge and decision-support that enhance the quality, safety, and efficiency of patient care; and (4) support of efficient processes for health care delivery. Critical building blocks of an EHR system are the electronic health records (EHR) maintained by providers (e.g., hospitals, nursing homes, ambulatory settings) and by individuals (also called personal health records)" (IOM, 2003).

[5] "An electronic Personal Health Record (ePHR) is a universally accessible, layperson comprehensible, lifelong tool for managing relevant health information, promoting health maintenance and assisting with chronic disease management via an interactive, common data set of electronic health information and e-health tools. The ePHR is owned, managed, and shared by the individual or his or her legal proxy(s) and must be secure to protect the privacy and confidentiality of the health information it contains. It is not a legal record unless so defined and is subject to various legal limitations" (Healthcare Information and Management Systems Society, 2005).

tions and disparate information systems, including data from laboratories, pharmacies, plans, physicians, or hospitals. A major benefit of eHealth is the opportunity it offers doctors and other health care providers to connect with the patient through these systems.

Neither patients nor the health care system can benefit, however, unless the new health information technology is actually adopted and used. Adoption rates for electronic health records in solo practitioner offices are about 13 percent, while in large medical practices adoption rates are somewhere between 19 percent to 57 percent. Overall the adoption rate for EHRs in physician offices is between 17 percent and 25 percent. For hospitals, the adoption rates for EHRs range from 16 percent to 59 percent. CPOE system adoption rates for hospitals range from 4 percent to 21 percent.

According to a Pew Internet and American Life research study, 79 percent of Internet users, or 95 million American adults, have searched online for information on at least one major health topic (Fox, 2006). A more recent Pew survey indicated that adults living with a disability or chronic disease are less likely than others to go online, but once they are online, they are more likely to look for health information (Fox, 2007). Such consumer use of electronic systems for obtaining health information illustrates the potential value of consumer-facing Health IT applications.

According to an October 2005 research report supported by the Markle Foundation, 60 percent of Americans support the creation of a secure online "personal health record" service that would allow consumers to

- check and refill prescriptions;
- get results over the Internet;
- check for mistakes in the medical record; and
- conduct secure and private e-mail communication with your doctor or doctors (Markle Foundation, 2005).

In a recent Commonwealth Fund survey of consumer views about key health care issues, 94 percent of respondents felt that having easy access to medical records was very or somewhat important and 93 percent felt the doctors having access to their medical records was very or somewhat important (Shoen et al., 2006). In June 2006, when the eHealth Initiative Foundation conducted a number of focus groups and a phone survey of individuals in the Gulf Coast area on the topic of electronic health information exchange, it found that 70 percent of those individuals favored secure, electronic health information exchange that is "protected and exchanged under current medical privacy and confidentiality standard procedures" (Shea et al., 2007).

In recent years there has been an increasing interest in consumer-facing applications, with very large corporations such as Microsoft and Google developing a number of applications in this area. Most efforts are, however, provider-centric initiatives, increasingly led by hospitals and are designed to exchange data across organizations. There is also some activity with health plans. Of particular value in what is occurring across the field of health information technology is connecting consumer applications with those that exchange clinical data.

The eHealth Initiative Foundation conducts an annual survey of Information Exchange Initiatives. The fourth annual survey of health information exchange at the state, regional, and community levels, conducted in 2007, found that of the 130 initiatives responding to the survey, 20 were at the beginning stages of effort (stage 1 or 2—see Table 2-1 for

TABLE 2-1 Seven-Stage Framework for Assessing and Tracking the Development of Health Information Exchange Initiatives at the State and Local Levels

Stage	Description
Stage 1	Recognition of the need for health information exchange among multiple stakeholders in your state, region or community. (Public declaration by a coalition or political leader)
Stage 2	Getting organized; defining shared vision, goals, and objectives; identifying funding sources, setting up legal and governance structures. (Multiple, inclusive meetings to address needs and frameworks)
Stage 3	Transferring vision, goals and objectives to tactics and business plan; defining your needs and requirements; securing funding. (Funded organizational efforts under sponsorship)
Stage 4	Well under way with implementation—technical, financial, and legal. (Pilot project or implementation with multiyear budget identified and tagged for a specific need)
Stage 5	Fully operational health information organization; transmitting data that is being used by health care stakeholders.
Stage 6	Fully operational health information organization; transmitting data that is being used by health care stakeholders and have a sustainable business model.
Stage 7	Demonstration of expansion of organization to encompass a broader coalition of stakeholders than present in the initial operational model.

Reprinted with permission from the eHealth Initiative and Foundation for eHealth Initiative, 2008c. *Results of 2008 Survey on Health Information Exchange: State of the Field.* http://www.ehealthinitiative.org/HIESurvey/2008StateOfTheField.mspx.

description of stages), 68 were in the process of implementation (stage 3 or 4), 32 were operational (stage 5, 6, or 7), 5 were no longer moving forward, and 5 organizations did not respond to the stage of development question. Thirty of the initiatives that responded to the 2006 survey reported advances in their stage of development (eHealth Initiative and Foundation for eHealth Initiative, 2008b). While some of these initiatives have not been successful, there are a number that have progressed well. At the same time, there are more efforts directed at consumer-facing applications, which is an entirely different model from the provider-centric initiatives.

Congress has introduced bills over the last several years that were intended to address key barriers to health IT adoption. During 2007 more than 19 bills related to health IT were introduced both in the House and Senate, most notably the Wired for Health Care Quality Act of 2007 (S. 1693), approved by the U.S. Senate Committee on Health, Education, Labor, and Pensions in August 2007, and a companion bill introduced in the House in early October 2007, both of which include several provisions related to health IT (Marchibroda, 2008).

The Department of Health and Human Services (HHS) has also played a leadership role in moving the health IT agenda forward by emphasizing its four cornerstones of value-driven health care which are to

- adopt interoperable health information technology (health IT standards);
- measure and publish quality information (quality standards);
- measure and publish price information (price standards); and
- promote quality and efficiency of care (incentives) (HHS, 2006).

The HHS Office of the National Coordinator for Health Information Technology has made a number of efforts aimed at health IT standards harmonization, standards certification, and trial implantation of health IT prototypes. More work remains to be accomplished, however, particularly in the area of modifying payment strategies to reward those health IT initiatives that are accomplishing more rather than just doing more. A number of individual states have also gotten involved, with executive orders and legislative activities at the state level.

Marchibroda concluded that, given the momentum of health IT, it is now a time of tremendous opportunity to develop eHealth systems that can address health literacy issues. At the same time, if such issues are not attended to, the creation of eHealth and health information applications may actually exacerbate existing problems, rather than providing a mechanism to help solve them.

SKILLS ESSENTIAL FOR eHEALTH

Cameron D. Norman, Ph.D.
Assistant Professor, Department of Public Health Sciences,
University of Toronto

Since the 1960s and early 1970s there has been a shift from provider-centered care to consumer-centered care, with individuals being encouraged to search for answers themselves and to take greater responsibility for their own health. This has resulted in the growth of consumer-directed material, such as self-help books and Internet websites.

Health information is known to be an essential component of health behavior change. People must have information about the threat, the opportunity, and the ability to make decisions about what actions to take. With the rise of the Internet and the World Wide Web, the public now has access to the greatest information tool ever available, with individuals able to obtain a great deal of medical information on health at a distance, without having to see a practitioner. So far, however, there are no established guidelines for how to use the Internet or how to produce content for it.

The Pew Internet and American Life Project (Fox, 2007) found that more than 80 percent of Internet users report seeking health information online; for Internet users with chronic conditions, the rate is 86 percent. And those percentages will most likely increase over the coming years. Unfortunately, few check the sources of information thoroughly and while there is widespread availability of health resources online, a search engine is usually the starting point. Thus, consumers need to have skills to effectively seek out the desired information, evaluate it, and then apply the information they find toward solving their health problems. More than half (58 percent) of those who report searching for online health information also report that the information they found affected their health decisions, and 39 percent say the information they found changed the way that they cope with a chronic condition or manage pain (Fox, 2006, 2007). Given these data, it is clear that it would be valuable to provide individuals with skills essential for eHealth.

Robert Logan maintains that the Internet and networked tools for health represent a fundamentally new form of language that requires a new form of literacy (Logan, 2000). A quick search for information on the common cold can be used to illustrate the difficulties in eHealth literacy.

A search of WebMD (www.webmd.com) for information on the common cold produces a page with a great deal of text and advertisements for a variety of products, not all of which are related to the health condition described on the page. At the bottom of the text-heavy page is a list of potential treatments. To one with low literacy, such a page of information can be quite intimidating.

Another site with health information was hosted by the Canadian Health Network (www.canadianhealthnetwork.ca), a federation of different health resources that does not produce all of the health materials itself.[6] If one searched the Canadian Health Network for information on the common cold, one was actually taken to another site—Capital Health, which is located in Edmonton, Canada. While information obtained in this redirected manner might be accurate and appropriate, an automatic switch of sites can be confusing to consumers who expect one site and get another.

If one goes to www.healthfinder.gov, a site sponsored by the U.S. Department of Health and Human Services, and types in "cold," one is presented with a page listing a variety of options to click for information. Clicking on an option then takes the user to a PDF (portable document format) file that provides information about the cold. A PDF file, however, requires the user to have Adobe Acrobat Reader which, if one does not have the software, must be downloaded. A person with minimal eHealth skills may be confused about what to do, and wonder why it is that a piece of software must be downloaded to the computer in order to read the page of information. Such actions can be frightening for those unfamiliar with health information or working with computers.

Finally, if one seeks information about the common cold from NHS Direct (www.nhsdirect.nhs.uk), the website of the National Health Service in the United Kingdom, one finds the design of the site to be fairly pleasing to the eye. The page on the common cold is uncluttered, although there is a fair amount of text and there are also some links for basic terms such as sneeze, lungs, and larynx that can be used to look up additional information. Nonetheless, despite its clear design, the site demands more than basic literacy to understand and therefore can be a challenge for those with low literacy skills and involves more than basic literacy.

As these examples illustrate, there are challenges to using the Internet for obtaining health information. In response to such challenges, the concept of eHealth literacy has been developed. eHealth literacy is "the ability to seek, find, understand, and appraise health information from electronic sources and apply the knowledge gained to addressing or solving a health problem" (Norman and Skinner, 2006b) Such a definition is consistent with Logan's contentions that use of the Internet is complex and its use plus the use of other networked tools constitutes a new lan-

---

[6] The Canadian Health Network was operating at the time of this workshop, however it has since ceased operations. Therefore, the example provided during this presentation can no longer be accessed.

guage form and requires a new set of skills to fully understand it (Logan, 2000). The eHealth literacy definition is framed in terms of action because if one is looking for information about a health problem, one is looking not just for information but for actions that one can take in order to solve a health problem.

Two types of skills are needed for eHealth: general skills and specific skills. General skills apply to a number of different contexts and settings and include traditional literacy (reading, writing, and numeracy), media literacy (media analysis skills), and information literacy (information seeking and understanding). Specific skills include such things as computer literacy (IT skills), health literacy (health knowledge comprehension), and science literacy (science process and outcome).

Four out of 10 Americans and Canadians have low literacy, making it difficult for them to function in everyday society (Rubenson et al., 2007; Statistics Canada, 2005). Thus in the case of eHealth interventions that are largely text-based, 4 out of every 10 people who might benefit from the intervention will have a great deal of difficulty reading the material. In the case of mathematical literacy (numeracy), one-quarter of U.S. 15-year-olds scored at or below the lowest proficiency level (Miller et al., 2007). To the extent that eHealth involves simple mathematical calculations such as addition or subtraction, or an understanding of numbers, those with low numeracy skills will likely find it difficult to understand the information presented. Such individuals will also have difficulty reading maps or understanding simple charts.

Media literacy refers to the skills necessary to think critically and to act based on information from media-based messages. Media literacy places information in a social and political context and considers issues such as the marketplace, audience relations, and the role of the medium in the message. Those with low media literacy lack awareness of bias or perspective in media pronouncements, both in terms of what is presented and what is not presented. They also have difficulty understanding that the media has both explicit and implied messages and they have difficulty deriving meaning from media messages.

The third general skill involved in eHealth literacy, information literacy, involves a more general understanding of information. An information literate person knows "how knowledge is organized, how to find information, and to use information in a way that others can learn from them" (American Library Association Presidential Committee on Information Literacy, 1989). Those with low information literacy are unable to see connections between information from multiple sources such as books, pamphlets, and websites. They are, therefore, unable to understand that one may have to triangulate pieces of information from various sources to build an entire picture of the subject about which they are seeking information. Those with low information literacy are also unfamiliar with local libraries and other repositories of information, and they are unable to frame search questions in a manner that produces desired results.

As described above, the specific skills involved in eHealth include computer literacy, science literacy, and health literacy. Computer literacy is a general awareness of and skill in using computer-based technology to solve problems (Logan, 2000). It relates both to computers and to the kind of technologies that surround the use of computers, such as the use of a keyboard, mouse, or printer. As Skinner and colleagues point out, computer literacy involves more than simply access to this type of technology; it is also about relative access and the comfort with which one accesses computers (Skinner et al., 2003a, 2003b). For example, Canada was the first country in the world to connect each of its public schools to the Internet. One might therefore say that all Canadian students have access to the Internet. But if access is only at certain times of the day, or in one particular room where the teacher is present and overseeing what students are doing, a young person wanting to find information on sexual health may find it difficult to do so.

Science literacy, another skill necessary for eHealth, is an understanding of the nature, aims, methods, application, limitations and politics of creating knowledge in a systematic manner (Laugksch, 2000). Research on scientific literacy suggests that only 17 percent of Americans are considered able to understand basic science (Gross, 2006). This means that the remaining 83 percent of Americans lack an understanding of the cumulative, dynamic nature of scientific knowledge. They are not aware that science can be understood and used by non-scientists, and they are unfamiliar with simple science terminology, the process of discovery, or how scientific knowledge is translated into practice. Yet 87 percent of online users (128 million adults) use the Internet as a research tool, and 70 percent have used the Internet to look up a scientific term (Horrigan, 2006).

Finally, eHealth demands health literacy skills. The Pew Internet and American Life Project found that 64 percent of Americans had searched online for health information in 1 of 17 areas[7] identified by the Pew Internet and American Life Project (Fox, 2006). Seventy-three percent of

---

[7] The 17 areas are specific disease or medical problem (64%); certain medical treatment or procedure (51%); diet, nutrition, vitamins, or nutritional supplements (49%); exercise or fitness (44%); prescription or over-the-counter drugs (37%); a particular doctor or hospital (29%); health insurance (28%); alternative treatments or medicines (22%); depression, anxiety, stress, or mental health issues (22%); environmental health hazards (22%); experimental treatments or medicines (18%); immunizations or vaccinations (16%); dental health information (15%); Medicare or Medicaid (13%); sexual health information (11%); how to quit smoking (9%); and problems with drugs or alcohol (8%).

individuals with a chronic condition have searched online for information and those with chronic conditions were more likely than others to report that the results of an online search influenced their health and care behavior related to their condition (Fox, 2007). Yet those with low health literacy[8] have difficulty following simple self-care directions or prescription instructions. They fear taking medications without assistance and are unfamiliar with or lack understanding of basic health care terms.

As can be seen from this discussion, a number of skills are necessary to successfully navigate the eHealth arena. Identifying these skills and understanding the extent to which individuals possess these skills should help in the design of better eHealth tools and systems. The eHealth literacy scale (eHEALS) (Norman and Skinner, 2006a) was developed in order to provide a concise measure of a patient's self-perceived skill and comfort in using information technology for health. It contains 10 questions, graded on a 5-point Likert scale with the questions designed to measure knowledge of existing eHealth resources, how to find resources, how to evaluate resources, how to use resources, and how to apply eHealth resources to health problems. eHEALS has been tested in both intervention trials and population health surveys with multicultural samples. It has shown excellent internal consistency (scale alpha = .89-.97) and has good test-retest reliability. The scale is publicly available (http://www.jmir.org/2006/4/e27), has been translated into multiple languages, and is currently in use in 10 countries.

eHealth literacy is growing in importance. Consumer-directed electronic tools are transforming the way that consumers receive information—for good and for bad. Blogs,[9] wikis,[10] and a number of what are called Web 2.0[11] technologies allow people with little skill in programming to post information on line. This in turn means that the amount of information, including health information, found on the Internet is coming at a faster rate and from more diverse sources than ever. Unfortunately, there is no overall mechanism for monitoring and assessing the reliability of that

---

[8] It is estimated that 90 million Americans have low health literacy, that is, trouble understanding and acting on health information (IOM, 2004).

[9] "A blog is a website where entries are made in journal style and displayed in a reverse chronological order. Blogs often provide commentary or news on a particular subject, such as food, politics, or local news; some function as more personal online diaries" (Sussex Learning Network, 2006).

[10] A wiki "is a website that allows multiple users to create, modify and organize web page content in a collaborative manner" (Governors State University, 2008).

[11] Web 2.0 is "a term often applied to a perceived ongoing transition of the World Wide Web from a collection of websites to a full-fledged computing platform serving web applications to end users. It refers to a supposed second-generation of Internet-based services—such as social networking sites, wikis, communication tools, and folksonomies—that emphasize online collaboration and sharing among users" (2020 Systems).

information, which makes it particularly important to provide the public with eHealth literacy skills.

eHealth literacy is not just a static, objective assessment of whether or not an individual is literate. It is something that will change as technology changes. It is a process of learning, not just an outcome, so eHealth literacy levels will constantly be in flux as technology changes. As Marshall McLuhan once said, the medium really is the message, and it is true here. Literacy skills are related to the medium in which they are applied. These skills are teachable, but they require constant remediation and updating.

STRATEGIES FOR RAISING HEALTH LITERACY IN ARIZONA MEDICAID MEMBERS: NEW APPROACHES FOR STATE MEDICAID "HEALTH KNOWLEDGE BUILDERS"

Anthony Rodgers
Director, Arizona Health Care Cost Containment System

"Health literacy is one of the most widespread obstacles to achieving better health outcomes in the United States" (AgrAbility Project, 2005) but eHealth technology can help address this issue. Medicaid enrolls what are probably the most vulnerable, least educated individuals in the country, and many of these individuals have mental health diseases and other chronic illnesses that hinder them from effectively participating in the health care delivery system. Additionally, Medicaid usually sees these individuals at a point of medical crisis. Arizona's Medicaid program, the Arizona Health Care Cost Containment System (AHCCCS), has a fourfold vision

- to encourage informed, active patients interacting with informed clinical teams;
- to have a medical home[12] for each individual that is capable of understanding each patient;
- to have a single view of each patient through electronic health records; and
- to have clinical decision support tools.

---

[12] A medical home "is not just a building, house or hospital, but a team approach to providing health care. A Medical Home originates in a primary health care setting that is family-centered and compassionate. A partnership develops between the family and the primary health care practitioner. Together they access all medical and non-medical services needed by the child and family to achieve maximum potential. The Medical Home maintains a centralized, comprehensive record of all health related services to promote continuity of care" (Colorado Department of Public Health and Environment, 2008).

To achieve this vision requires a transformation of the Arizona Medicaid health care system. Necessary components of this transformation will include the widespread adoption of interoperable health information technology (HIT), electronic health information exchange, and electronic health records that are transferable and transportable either through the patient or through electronic means. Furthermore, there must be greater use of Web-based clinical and patient decision-support tools that use a common health data set and evidence-based references. Such a system would enable Medicaid to use the data in its files to provide clinical decision tools that allow physicians to see the individual patient episode of care or care plan and also make it possible for AHCCCS to aggregate this information for a broader perspective of the health of the Medicaid population. Finally, the system needs internet and communication tools that support the delivery of personalized health information and health literacy competency for Medicaid beneficiaries.

Ratzan and Parker defined health literacy as "the degree to which individuals have the capacity to obtain, process, and understand basic health information and services needed to make appropriate health decisions" (Ratzan and Parker, 2000). Improving health literacy levels will help create informed and activated AHCCCS members. To design interventions aimed specifically at improving health literacy, AHCCCS identified several skill sets inherent in the broad definition of health literacy. One such set of skills is functional health literacy skills, the basic reading and writing skills necessary to understand and follow simple health information. Another skill set is interactive health literacy skills which are more advanced than basic skills and include the ability to interact with a system that is providing personalized health information, not just general health information. This set also includes the cognitive and interpersonal skills needed and the confidence necessary for interacting or partnering with a clinical professional.

Critical thinking skills are another component of health literacy. These skills involve the ability to analyze and make value-based choices when presented with alternative possibilities—the choice between medications with different side effects, for example, or the choice of surgery versus longer-term medical intervention. Finally, there are focused health literacy skills that are more specialized and that involve the knowledge and ability to engage in consumer-directed care by performing defined patient self-care management support tasks and wellness activities. These skills will be increasingly important as people move more into home-based and community-based care.

AHCCCS has a Medicaid Transformation Grant to develop new eHealth tools to improve health literacy. During Phase I of the grant, the objective will be to reconfigure available technology. This will be accomplished by building electronic health records, devising patient-decision support tools, providing Internet messaging capabilities for both clinicians and beneficiaries, developing Web multi-media health education efforts, and devising e-learning programs in multiple languages that will, over time, help document improvements in health literacy.

Phase II of the grant involves Web-based interactive games and personalized educational programming (seen as a particularly valuable way to reach adolescents and children), Internet-connected biometric monitoring devices (intended to keep more people at home and in community-based services), and Web 2.0 (Web-based health and human service support networking) that will be used to create self-support groups among different populations.

Figure 2-1 below illustrates the infrastructure transformation toward which AHCCCS is working. The enabling technologies are the health information exchange infrastructure, electronic health record infrastructure, the Web-based e-learning programming infrastructure, and the knowledge building and transfer infrastructure. With properly configured enabling technologies creating the processes through which the various Medicaid programs (e.g., acute care, long-term care, disease-management health education, and population-based education) operate, the end result is a transformed health system. Once the connection exists, new products and tools can be added and rapidly deployed.

The major issue is getting the infrastructure in place to transform the

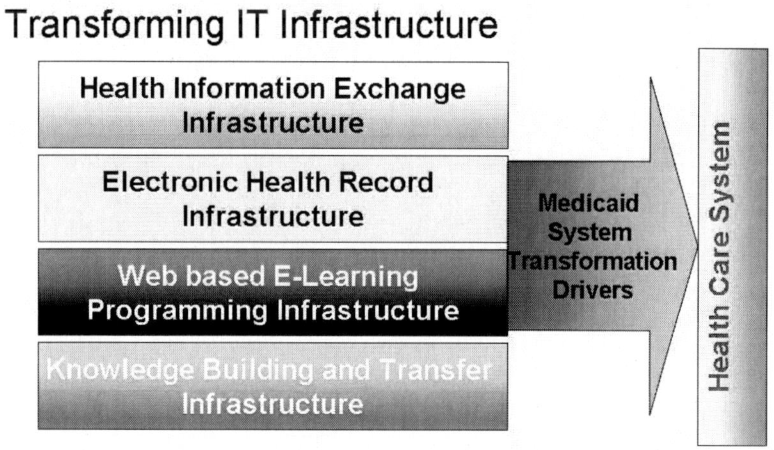

Transforming IT Infrastructure

- Health Information Exchange Infrastructure
- Electronic Health Record Infrastructure
- Web based E-Learning Programming Infrastructure
- Knowledge Building and Transfer Infrastructure

→ Medicaid System Transformation Drivers → Health Care System

FIGURE 2-1 eHealth infrastructure of Medicaid system transformation.
SOURCE: Rodgers, 2008.

system. What AHCCCS is attempting is to integrate the system virtually—to integrate it with information and to integrate more rapid deployment of knowledge—which should result in improved quality and reduced costs. In such a system one would have the same information reference points no matter where one was located—in a community clinic, a physician's office, or elsewhere.

Phase I will include a focus on interactive multimedia product development that goes beyond static health content. Such products will include e-learning modules, electronic health assessments, Web-based health coaching, Web-logs, streaming video,[13] Web-based health awareness campaigns, eHealth-connected provider offices for access to downloadable personalized health videos, and podcasts.

Multimedia education will focus first on raising the health literacy of those with chronic diseases and, in particular, will be aimed at helping individuals understand their chronic illnesses. Over time the materials will address other important conditions and situations of relevance for the AHCCCS population, for example, how to keep one's health care coverage in place and how to use one's health plan.

eHealth education will be personalized. The information that a person retains from an educational program is dependent upon a number of factors including to whom that individual relates well and who is providing the education. In many education efforts the same product is delivered in the same way by the same person. AHCCCS's goal is to deliver education in a much more personal and culturally sensitive manner, tailoring the important content of that education to the various needs of the population and using messengers who are similar to and can relate to members of various populations. Additionally, these multimedia education programs will be developed in English, Spanish, and in some cases Native American languages.

AHCCCS strategies for building eHealth literacy products include knowledge-building programming capability and rapid production of e-learning programs with multiple content sources. The rapid production goal for AHCCCS staff is to produce a new program every day. If it takes 2 months to develop and deliver each audio or video program, that is too long. In a rapid production cycle, content is duplicated but it is delivered by a different person and is aimed at a different population. One can do a great deal with today's camcorders and digital equipment. One does not need a $100,000 studio; one needs just a couple of creative people with a camera. To establish that the programs actually work, innovation centers,

---

[13] A streaming video is a "one-way video transmission over a data network. It is widely used on the Web as well as company networks to play video clips and video broadcasts" (Techweb, 2008).

established by AHCCCS at federally qualified health centers with volunteer physicians, will be test sites for product prototypes.

AHCCCS has recently introduced a website. One of the things of interest is who will access the website. Table 2-2 below provides an overview of utilization trends for 1 month this year.

The AHCCCS basic website is called My Arizona Health and Wellness (www.myazhealthandwellness.com). The mission of the website is "to build health and wellness literacy in AHCCCS members so that they make decisions that improve their health care quality and reduce preventable health care care costs through the utilization of interactive, personalized health education and health literacy competency" (Rodgers, 2008). This website is the basic mechanism that will be used to deliver many of the eHealth tools AHCCCS will develop. The website also supports the governor's executive order (Napolitano, 2008) to reduce the escalation of health care costs for Arizona by the following

- reducing costs through patient-centered care that integrates wellness, prevention, self-care education and chronic disease management;

TABLE 2-2 Snapshot of Web Utilization Trends/Data January 2008 to February 2008

Website	Healthwise Knowledgebase Content Usage	
Site Usage: - 1,152 visits - 897 (72%) absolute unique visits	Top 10 Search Terms: Pneumonia Asthma Dental BOOK-n873	Top 10 Topic Views: Women's Health Interactive Tools Health Eating Men's Health

Top Traffic Sources:
- 79% referring site
  (AHCCCS website)
- 18% direct traffic
	(surgery-carpal
	  tunnel syndrome)
	Cancer
	Diabetes
	COPD
		Pregnancy
		Children's Health
		Diabetes
		Depression
		Pneumonia

Top Content visits: - Health Resources - Get Covered, Stay Covered - Wellness in Arizona	BOOK-d904 (surgery-varicose veins) Immunizations Dairy	Type 2 Diabetes
E-mail signups: 40 (mostly internal/staff)	Healthwise Content Usage: 651 visits Hits: 19,722 Visit duration by minutes: Majority (0-1 minute)	

SOURCE: Rodgers, 2008.

- implementing new incentives and policy changes for providers to adopt e-health technologies and evidence-based standards; and
- improving accountability by empowering consumers with quality, cost and health information.

It is important that each beneficiary have an e-mail address and access to the internet so that each person can obtain needed information and also so that eHealth tools can be used effectively. One of AHCCCS's requirements will be that each beneficiary have an e-mail address and, eventually, that each individual document how he or she will access the Internet. If an individual does not have a way to access the internet, then AHCCCS will take responsibility for devising a way to provide access. Such options could include using cell phones, text messaging, or an iPod or MP3 player on which information can be downloaded.

One new tool that can be used for patient Internet access in a provider's office is the "Tablet," a handheld personal computer with an 8.4 inch screen that runs Microsoft Windows XP. AHCCCS envisions a time when each patient who enters a physician's office will be handed a device that provides access to the Internet. The patient will then be asked to update his or her health history (AHCCCS is developing a Web-based health history), and each patient will also access his or her personal health account which will contain a personalized audio/video file of e-learning programs.

In this future vision, once a patient accesses his or her personal health account, the physician will be able to view the information and make sure that the patient understood the individual e-learning programs, since patient responses will be automatically uploaded to the electronic health record (EHR). If misunderstandings occur, the physician will then be able to correct the information and discuss the problems further.

This is the vision of "medical home" that each AHCCCS beneficiary will eventually have. To become a medical home, primary and specialty sites will be required to have EHRs, Internet connectivity, an AHCCCS Health Education Kiosk or Wi-Fi[14]-enabled touch-screen tablet, and a high-definition television with speakers in the examination room so that patients can access the e-learning tools. These e-learning programs will not be something that the patient obtains from the Web, but rather will be programs developed specifically for the chronic conditions or other problems

---

[14] "Wi-Fi (short for 'wireless fidelity') is a term for certain types of wireless local area network (WLAN) that use specifications in the 802.11 family. The term Wi-Fi was created by an organization called the Wi-Fi Alliance, which oversees tests that certify product interoperability. A product that passes the alliance tests is given the label 'Wi-Fi certified' (a registered trademark)" (SearchMobileComputing.com, 2008).

the patient has. Physicians will be familiar with the programs and so will be able to engage in a dialogue with each patient about his or her specific conditions, using the e-learning programs as a basis for discussion.

In one AHCCCS video on diabetes, the main character is a white adult male talking about diabetes while standing next to his vehicle in a parking lot. The video presentation was made by Knowledge Builders, the name that members of the AHCCCS staff gave themselves. The next character featured in a video with the same content might be an adult female Hispanic who is Spanish-speaking or perhaps an adult male Spanish-speaking individual or a Native American–speaking individual. In the AHCCCS approach, Rodgers stated, the same content is used for everyone, but the content is delivered by different characters depending on the audience. The purpose is to see if this engages the various beneficiary populations. Rapid production of these materials allows change in the material. AHCCCS evaluates its e-learning programs to determine exactly who is learning what and where most of the problems are. Material is then edited to address identified problems.

Rodgers concluded by predicting that AHCCCS eHealth, properly configured, will help address one of the major obstacles to achieving better outcomes, that is, eHealth literacy.

DISCUSSION

George Isham, M.D., M.S.
HealthPartners
Moderator

One questioner asked Rodgers to provide more detail about the infrastructure that AHCCCS is building. Rodgers replied that the first effort is being directed at EHRs so that providers will be able to exchange health information. This is not an EHR in the fullest sense, he said, but it will include the problem list, information regarding medications, lab results, x-ray views, and clinical notes. Further down the road the idea is to be able to embed files and other information into the EHR. The e-learning programming for patient-focused education will be available through the Web, as will be provider-focused education, the clinical support tools, and the patient decision-support tools. These will be configured with the EHR.

Another audience member asked whether AHCCCS is educating consumers about the system as it is being developed. Are they learning what eHealth means, what an electronic medical system can do, and how to use the specific hardware (e.g., the tablet discussed earlier)? Rodgers replied that the system is not currently in the market and available. What does exist is a prototype that is being tested. Once this is validated and additional models are developed, AHCCCS plans to hold focus sessions with various groups to determine if different populations engage the system differently and if individuals can relate to the system.

The assumption is that the system will work, but that needs to be validated. Once validated, the idea is to use the innovation centers discussed earlier as the first beta sites. There are several options that one might use in these sites, including a workstation-type kiosk or provision of the tablets. One could also create an education room, but since AHCCCS plans to ultimately offer these services in provider offices where space tends to be limited, creating a separate education room may not be the best option to pursue. The hope is that access will eventually be available in the homes. The most logical access point, however, is the physician offices where patients can use the system at the time of their appointment. This is probably also the time at which the patients will be most motivated to seek information, and it will be a good way to use waiting time.

Norman was asked to comment on what is involved in teaching individuals to be computer literate. Norman responded that there is a complex and a simple way to teach computer literacy. The simple approach is usually constructed around a particular piece of technology, such as e-mail. In this case, one works with the individual to find the simplest route to e-mail and puts an icon on the desktop computer so that it is a simple matter to call up the e-mail. The idea is to have a familiar entry screen so that use is simple.

eHealth is a place, although most do not think of it that way, Norman continued. It is a place to go in the system. A system needs benchmarks or landmarks that are easily associated with where the individual using the system needs to go. One should have a set of screens with a consistent style throughout the application, and people must be trained to understand the screens in order to use the system.

The more complex problem arises when one is attempting to teach people to search for information, that is when the people will need to use multiple platforms. Just as is the case with learning to speak another language, it is not something one can pick up in a weekend course; it is a much more complex task. A constant dialogue is needed, with markers for learning the language of computers and information searching. The key is to find where individuals are in terms of their knowledge and comfort levels. That is what eHEALS is designed to do.

Rodgers added that individuals must also have a reason to want to use the technology. If they are not interested, if they do not perceive the value of using the system, they will not use it. By grabbing individuals' attention with what one might think of as medical entertainment or with something that is fun and real to them, it becomes much easier to get them to want to use the technology.

Another questioner asked Rodgers, what happens when one is dealing with multiple chronic conditions since people seem to be able to understand only three concepts at any one time? Individuals need to be able to do many things, not just three, both in terms of navigating technology and in terms of self-management. Clinical professionals may identify specific things that they think are most important for such individuals to know. Conversely, those from the technological or navigational side might identify another set of skills. How can one deliver the right information at the right time to the right person so that that person is doing the right thing?

Rodgers responded that AHCCCS is ready to learn from its beneficiaries what works best for them and what does not work. The system must be modular, and it must be engaging, interesting, and real-world relevant to those using it. When one is working with Native Americans, for example, the programs and the person delivering them must understand the conditions (e.g., nutrition, daily life, etc.) in which that population operates and what strategies they might be willing to employ.

The key to being able to make such an approach work is technology, as technology is very forgiving and flexible, and it allows one to make relatively inexpensive changes as conditions change. With technology there is a great deal of flexibility, much more so than with the static pamphlet approach.

One questioner stated that quite a bit of research has been conducted that is relevant to AHCCCS's idea of delivering health information to people in a kiosk environment—for example, on such things as where the kiosks are located and whether people enjoy using them. A number of studies have shown that, for reasons that may or may not apply to Arizona's plan, using kiosks generally does not work well.

Despite that, the questioner continued, what Rodgers describes appears to be a promising approach, and she said that she is particularly interested in the idea of focus groups and what individuals actually learn from the e-learning programs. The National Library of Medicine has illustrative tutorials on its Medline Plus in both Spanish and English. These are very popular with those with low health literacy and with those who work with such populations. It would be interesting to see whether these could be made even more effective if they were delivered, as AHCCCS intends to do, by individuals who look or appear to be like those for whom the tutorials are designed, although in the case of some of the interactive materials illustrations rather than live individuals are used.

Rodgers responded that with the technology AHCCCS uses, change can be made relatively inexpensively. One does not need to reinvent things, just to present the material differently. The innovation centers, federally qualified health centers that have multiple and different types of populations, will serve as the laboratory for testing to determine how various populations respond to the various programs. It will be possible to determine whether individuals learn better from people like themselves. It will even be possible to measure variables over time because each time the system is accessed there is a time stamp and information on what modules are being accessed.

One participant suggested that the public library is a good place for people to learn to use technology as well as to learn basic information about health. In the United States, public libraries are accessible to almost everyone. Furthermore, Arizona has a fantastic Arizona Health Information Network.

Another participant suggested that non-English-speaking populations may not generally begin their searches on home computers. She asked Rodgers whether anyone has looked at the health information searching behavior of this population, including how they use the public library. Are there community intermediaries that can help?

Rodgers responded that AHCCCS has looked at this issue and that there are a number of community organizations that are willing to cooperate with them, such as libraries and schools that are willing to give computer access to parents. To date, however, AHCCCS has not had any product to provide access to. Eventually access will be provided not only in the physicians' offices, the clinics, and the hospitals, but also in a number of other places as well.

The key is for individuals to know when and for what they should access the internet. AHCCCS wants to have its beneficiaries fill out a health assessment as soon as they become eligible for services. Ultimately, the idea is to put the application online so that as they apply, they also fill out a health assessment form which will immediately provide information to the health plan that has never before been available.

One participant said that she sees health literacy as patient-centric. Most eHealth initiatives, however, appear to be provider-centric and motivated by costs. The main reason for increasing the efficiency of those systems appears to be recouping costs. At the Medicaid level, a very different system is driving eHealth. Here the issue is population health and how it can be improved, which is a more patient-centric approach. How can those motivated by costs be convinced to care about a patient-centric approach to eHealth?

Marchibroda responded that Rodgers' description of what is happening in Arizona makes her wish this was the case across the country. The reality is, however, that most current initiatives do not connect with the consumer. When one examines community-based initiatives, for example, only 4 percent are connecting with consumers. There are many barriers to connecting with consumers, including lack of a business case and concerns about liability, privacy, and confidentiality.

Out in the field, talking with leaders at the state, local, and national level about eHealth and health technology, people find that there is little awareness of the problems associated with low health literacy. The first step, then, must be an educational effort to raise awareness. Once awareness has been raised, efforts must focus on figuring out how to tackle the remaining issues.

Looking at the drivers of health IT, one might be able to make a business case for health literacy. In 2008, for example, analysts expect that $1.8 billion will be spent on chronic care management, most of which will be paid for by health plans or employers. Connecting consumers who have chronic conditions to e-learning systems built to address low health literacy issues—systems such as the one described by Rodgers—could offer a compelling business case for health literacy.

Another participant asked Rodgers how AHCCCS made the business case for developing its eHealth system and how it addressed issues of liability, privacy, and confidentiality. Rodgers responded that AHCCCS analyzed the potential return on investment and found that it is about $144 million a year. This is achieved on the provider side primarily through reduction of lab duplication, reduction in emergency room visits by providing patients with alternative sources of care, and reduction in x-rays by deploying images to where patients go for care.

On the consumer side the key element is compliance. There is significant variation in how well patients comply with physicians' instructions. It is difficult to see beyond the basic compliance issue because more data are needed—for example, data on whether patients are taking their medications. It is expected that the system will allow providers to track various kinds of compliance (e.g., whether patients pick up their medications or keep their health care appointments). Once data are available, personalized interventions can be developed—it will not work to implement the same intervention for everyone because the reasons for noncompliance are not uniform.

A participant asked if the speakers could elaborate on what Web 2.0 is. Norman responded that it reflects a shift in technology to more consumer-driven content. When the World Wide Web was first introduced, for example, in order to create a Web page, one had to know some programming language and HTML (HyperText Markup Language). With Web 2.0 technologies anyone, even those with no technical skill, can post on the Web with, for example a wiki (essentially an editable Web page) or a social networking Web page like Facebook. One does not need to understand any of the technology. Rodgers said that the great potential for health care is that patients with special health care needs can communicate with others who have the same needs, so that they can learn from each other. This is an entirely new way of providing coaching and obtaining support.

One participant pointed out that there is a movement called Health 2.0 which is focused on health. One Health 2.0 site, called Patients Like Me, allows patients to identify themselves, either anonymously or not, and then interact with others, describe their conditions, describe their experience with drugs, and so on. Patients Like Me also contains a variety of sites dedicated to particular health issues. For example, there is an ALS (amyotrophic lateral sclerosis) site within Patients Like Me.

One questioner referred to the study of CITL mentioned by Marchibroda which suggested that if standardized health care information were exchanged among health care IT systems, there would be a national savings of $86.8 billion. Is this a reasonable figure and how would that happen? Marchibroda responded that those conducting the study examined data flow across different organizations. The estimated savings come from a variety of things, such as reductions in duplicate lab tests and reductions in transactional costs related to messaging. In order to achieve the savings, one must provide multiple services to multiple parties in the system, which is not how things happen in the real health care system, in order to realize a return on the capital investment.

One participant stated that when she thinks of populations with low health literacy she thinks of recent immigrants, the elderly, and those with limited English proficiency. Would the tools that are being developed for eHealth actually disenfranchise these groups even more? How can these populations learn to use Health 2.0 or other eHealth tools? Won't these tools be of benefit only for other populations, those who do not have the health literacy problems faced by these disadvantaged populations?

Rodgers responded that, for AHCCCS efforts, the strategy is to keep eHealth tools really simple (e.g., point and click on pictures, not words) and to provide an easy set of audio/video instructions for those experiencing difficulty. To ensure that these tools are effective, one must start at the point of those being served and provide help, whether that is in the library or the physicians' offices. Even as more and more of the population becomes comfortable with using eHealth tools, there will still be a group for which using the tools will be a challenge. For these individuals, new strategies will need to be developed. The idea is to try something, evaluate what has been tried, learn from that evaluation about what works and what doesn't, and have a system that is flexible enough so that necessary changes can be made.

One participant observed that the role of individuals is going to be important in the realization of cost savings. Individuals will have to be literate enough to interact with the technology in order to harvest savings. How much of the projected $144 million for Arizona or the $86.6 billion estimate savings will depend upon computer literacy?

Norman responded that the eHealth system is dependent upon individuals with some type of literacy. The system must be structured in such a way that it meets the needs of those using it, that is, it must be user friendly for those with low health literacy or cultural needs. It cannot just repackage the same old information in a digital format. The design of the system must consider who is using it, how those using the system interact with technology, what their needs are generally (such as literacy and cultural needs), as well as what their needs are at a given time.

Rodgers said that one of the tools that will be important in the future is an iPod or iPod-like device that enables the user to download information. With such a tool individuals will not have to use a computer. Rather, they will need to understand how to record and then play back information. While such a mechanism is less interactive, it will still provide important health information to users.

One participant said that the focus in developing eHealth systems should not be just on the package of technological or system tools. Rather, it will be critical to recognize the importance of the skills that individuals bring to the table and to understand what it is one is asking people to do.

With the market driving development, competition is the name of the game: How can one do this a little cheaper, a little better? Medicaid in Arizona is doing it one way—and it seems to be a good way. Other health care organizations are developing different approaches. People using eHealth systems are confronted with 25 different ways of doing one thing. How can they possibly navigate through these options? What is needed is a system that people can navigate, one in which a set of skills can be taught and used throughout health care. While cost may be the driver, the real bottom-line quest is, Do these systems actually improve the health of the population?

3

Outcomes and Challenges of eHealth Approaches: Panel 1

INTERNET APPROACHES FOR eHEALTH IN LOW-LITERACY AND LIMITED-ENGLISH-PROFICIENCY POPULATIONS

Rita Kukafka, Dr.P.H., M.A.
Columbia University, Mailman School of Public Health

The Harlem Health Promotion Center (HHPC) is one of the 33 Prevention Research Centers[1] funded by the Centers for Disease Control and Prevention to conduct applied research into disease prevention. These research centers serve as a bridge between science and practice, and between academia and vulnerable communities, working with communities to identify areas of concern and to develop practical strategies to address these concerns.

Since 2004 the HHPC has been using the methods of participatory action research[2] to develop the Digital Partners in Health Project, a health portal designed to provide culturally-relevant health information and decision support to consumers with low literacy. Building the project required information about how people of color use technology and seek health information. Unfortunately, there is very little community-level

---

[1] Prevention Research Centers are "a network of academic researchers, public health agencies, and community members that conducts applied research in disease prevention and control" (CDC, 2008).

[2] "Participatory action research (PAR) is a method of research where creating a positive social change is the predominant driving force" (Seymour-Rolls and Hughes, 2000).

data about such use, although some national and regional data do exist. Furthermore, little is known about the extent to which people of color have access to, or interest in, using the Internet for health-related activities.

For these reasons researchers at the HHPC spent a significant amount of time collecting data using a random-digit-dial survey of 646 Harlem residents 18 years of age and older. The survey collected data on the use of and access to different types of technology as well as data on demographics, general health, and health-information-seeking behaviors. About 77 percent of responders said they had used a computer and 87 percent reported having friends or family who use the Internet. This is useful information for understanding diffusion of and normative support for technology use.

The survey also found that 68 percent of respondents had one or more computers at home and 57 percent used the Internet at home. For those who did not have a computer at home, 76 percent said they knew where a computer was publicly available. Sixty percent of respondents said that the most important problem in accessing the computer is overcrowding. Other problems in access were cost (2 percent), equipment problems (4 percent), location or transportation (8 percent), and hours of operation (13 percent). It is certainly true in Harlem that libraries have long lines waiting for access to the Internet. These data show that there is an interest in using technology.

An examination of the demographics of those surveyed reveals that younger people are more likely to use the Internet, that English-speakers are more likely to use the Internet than those whose first language is other than English, and that African-Americans are more likely to be Internet users than Hispanics and Latinos. The data also show that Internet users are more likely to have higher educational attainment, are more likely to be employed, and have higher incomes than those who do not use the Internet. Internet users also had a higher perceived self-health rating.

As the data in Table 3-1 show, Internet users are more able to find health information and have less difficulty understanding it than non-users. On the other hand, there is no significant difference between Internet users and non-users when asked if they bring up something they have seen or read with the doctor.

Survey participants were also asked where they went the last time they needed information on a health issue. Doctors were the main source of information for both Internet users (44 percent) and non-users (78 percent), although non-users were much more likely to go to their doctors for information. The major difference between the groups was that 39 percent of Internet users said that they went to the internet for health information, which implies that the Internet users go to the internet for health information almost as often as they go to their doctors.

PANEL 1

TABLE 3-1 Health Information Seeking by Current Internet Use

	Internet Users	Non-Users	P Value
"I have difficulty understanding a lot of the health information I read."	70 (21.2)	128 (42.0)	<0.0001
"When I read or hear something concerning my health care, I bring it up with my doctor."	274 (83.3)	272 (87.7)	0.1101
"It is hard to find good answers to my health questions and concerns."	90 (27.5)	142 (47.3)	<0.0001
"Very" or "Somewhat" confident in ability to get health advice OR confidence in ability to get health advice or information if needed	290 (88.2)	247 (80.7)	0.0096
Scale: (1) Very confident, (2) Somewhat confident, (3) Slightly confident, (4) Not confident at all.	Mean (SD) 1.53 (0.77)	Mean (SD) 1.75 (0.92)	0.0014

SOURCE: Kukafka, 2008.

Participants were also asked how much they trust health-related information obtained from different sources. Figure 3-1 displays their responses. As can be seen, health care professionals are rated as an extraordinarily credible source of information. A high percentage (71 percent) of Internet users also trust health-related information found on the Internet.

The data also show that 63 percent of those who go to the Internet search for health information about specific diseases. This seems to be the major motivator for people to exert the effort needed to access information on the Internet. Sixty-one percent of people who go to the Internet look for information on diet, nutrition, and fitness. Other types of information sought on the Internet by the Harlem respondents included medicines (44 percent); insurance, doctors, or hospitals (38 percent); mental health (22 percent); sexual health (26 percent); substance abuse (21 percent); and smoking cessation (14 percent).

In terms of barriers to Internet use, the study found that the responses for non-users about why they did not use the Internet were, in order of frequency: worry about pornography and fraud, followed by not wanting or needing the Internet; too expensive; no time; and too complicated and hard to understand. Non-users were also asked to indicate whether they agreed with a number of statements. The Internet:

- Would help them find out things easily—82 percent agree, 10 percent disagree
- Helps people keep in touch—79 percent agree, 11 percent disagree
- Is mostly entertainment—55 percent agree, 34 percent disagree
- I'm missing out by not using it—54 percent agree, 39 percent disagree
- Is a dangerous thing—51 percent agree, 41 percent disagree
- Is too expensive—50 percent agree, 31 percent disagree
- Is confusing, hard to use—38 percent agree, 29 percent disagree

The HHPC also used focus groups to gather information. The data that follow are from 6 of the 17 focus groups, 3 with Hispanic-speaking populations and three with English-speaking populations. Each group had 6 to 8 participants, and each person was asked to characterize himself as either Web user or non-user. Results from these focus groups indicate that both Web users and non-users consider the Internet to be a legitimate source of health information, even among those for whom the Internet was not the preferred source. Convenience of use was a major factor in the use of the Internet. Although participants reported enjoying the freedom that the Internet allowed, many said they had difficulty understanding

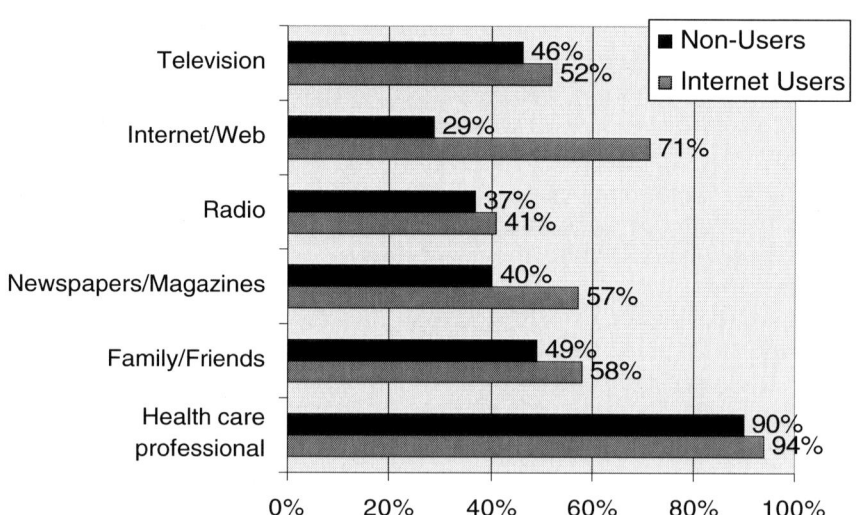

FIGURE 3-1 Trust in sources of health information.
SOURCE: Kukafka, 2008.

information found online and expressed a need for assistance in interpreting the health information.

One of the major barriers to seeking mainstream health information that the focus groups identified was suspicion and mistrust of the medical community, as illustrated with the following quotes: "I think one of the keys is that there is money involved. It is all about greed." "Those of us who are African-Americans are still grappling with the Tuskegee studies and the aftermath. So there are a lot of historical monsters with which we identify when it comes to medical community treatment and medical residents." "Then that leads me to conclude that there is just a lot of general information that we are not getting. There seems to be a mainstream level of information which gives you stuff to lead you into drugs, different things like that . . . there is like a whole stream of other viable alternatives that could work but you don't even hear about because it will blow all the mainstream drugs out." "The pharmaceutical companies are in bed with the FDA."

When members of the focus groups were asked what sources of information they trust, their answers included (ranked from most-mentioned to least-mentioned: their mothers; folk and alternative medicine ("grandmother's cures"); the health care provider; and, finally, the Internet. Everyone was aware of the importance of lifestyle, diet, and stress as contributors to health, but they expressed a general frustration with attempts to improve in these areas.

Using these data as background for understanding community attitudes, the HHPC project set out to build a Web portal[3] that Harlem residents would use. The conclusion was that the Web portal platform would need to do more than deliver health information, even if it were at a lower health literacy level, the portal would have to encourage a level of trust and cultural relevance as its foundation.

Developing the Web portal involves more than just developing content and images aimed at a particular literacy level. What HHPC realized is that the portal needs to facilitate an architecture of participation such as that found on Web 2.0, including such tools and services as blogs, RSS feeds,[4] and wikis. These different Internet instruments are examples of self-organizing structures where the principle of evolution will lead, in the course of time, to correct and complete content.

Table 3-2 provides a comparison of the principles of Web 2.0 tech-

---

[3] "A Web portal is a term, often used interchangeably with gateway, for a World Wide Web site whose purpose is to be a major starting point for users when they connect to the Web" (MariosAlexandrou.com, 2008).

[4] RSS (Really Simple Syndication) feed. "A syndication format that was developed by Netscape in 1999 and became very popular for aggregating updates to blogs and the news sites. RSS has also stood for 'Rich Site Summary'" (*PC Magazine*, 2008).

TABLE 3-2 Comparison of Principles of Web 2.0 and Web 1.0

Principle	Web 2.0	Traditional (Web 1.0)
Power	Decentralized (autonomy; information self sufficiency)	Centralized (experts); dependence
Priorities	Guided by community perspectives/norms, bottom up	Guided by technology developers
Filtering	Downstream (e.g., user ranking)	Upstream
Nature of information consumption	Coproducers	Passive receivers—consumption
Learning	Collective—capacity building	Exclusive
Content Credibility	Based on understandable language, experiential knowledge	Based on science
Culture	Enabling	Compliance

SOURCE: Kukafka, 2008.

nologies with the more traditional Web 1.0.[5] In moving from the Web 1.0 technology to Web 2.0 one moves from a centralized control situation to one of decentralized priorities. This is consistent with participatory action research methods, the methods used in the HHPC approach.

There are a number of mechanisms available in Web 2.0 by which the community filters material, such as community ratings. With Web 2.0 the receivers of information are coproducers of information as well, rather than just passive recipients, so that eventually, if enough people use the system, information is self-corrected. Content in Web 2.0 technologies is based on the experiential model or knowledge, and the culture of the technology moves from one of compliance to an enabling culture.

Web 2.0 structures facilitate social networking participation, collaboration, and openness within and between user groups. Information in this newer type of platform is liberated from the control of experts, which in the Harlem community was a source of mistrust. Community members will be able to create, assemble, organize, locate, and share content to meet their own needs and the needs of their community.

In a Web 2.0 technology, information is perceived as direct or unmediated. Such information is more credible than mediated information because the presence of mediation through a gatekeeper makes it pos-

---

[5] Web 1.0 is "a general reference to the World Wide Web during its first few years of operation. The term is mostly used to contrast the earlier days of the Web before blogs, wikis, social networking sites and Web-based applications became commonplace" (http://dictionary.zdnet.com/definition/Web+1.0.html). Accessed November 3, 2008.

sible to question the motives and intentions of the communicator (Stamm and Dube, 1994). A study by Baldry and colleagues showed that when health professionals actively encourage patients to view their own health records, it helps restore patient trust in the medical system (Baldry et al., 1986). Therefore, if the gatekeeper (e.g., the provider or hospital) moves out of the way and enables patients to view direct, unmediated information, that will improve the patients' level of trust in the provider.

As mentioned previously, the Digital Partners in Health project uses participatory action research (PAR) methods. The key goals of PAR are to produce knowledge and action that are directly useful to a group of people and to empower people at a second and deeper level through the process of constructing and using their own knowledge. Web 2.0 technologies can serve as an informatics approach to facilitate the principles and characteristics of PAR in disadvantaged populations. If one examines why PAR works, one finds that its principles are very similar to Web 2.0—that is, enabling the community itself to become part of the process, to communicate and participate, instead of using a closed technology driven by experts.

Developing the contents of the portal has involved a number of different types of individuals: technology developers, community people, informaticians, and public health people. There has been a great deal of negotiation among them about how much of the content on the portal will be unmediated (out of the control of experts) versus how much of it will be mediated. Some of the technology specifications, developed on the basis of user input, include the following

- Website content can be viewed by anyone but users must register to post or comment on the site's content.
- Registered users can:
  - submit their own blog (e.g., "How I quit smoking after ten failed attempts") or create special interest groups and social networks, each with its own discussion forums;
  - post events of interest, links to useful health resources, or participate in several special programs, such as the Harlem YMCA-sponsored Fitness Challenge; and
  - rate posts made by other users or flag posts as inappropriate (community policing and appraisal).
- An overall moderating team consisting of our experts as well as users will provide editorial control to ensure content quality.

The resulting website (gethealthyharlem.org) is not static. For example, there are RSS feeds of Harlem-specific health news where members can post comments and debate the news online. The website is not disease-driven; it is driven instead by determinants of health. Therefore it includes topics such as fitness, events, and spiritual concepts. Using empirical evidence about modifying health behavior and improving health outcomes, HHPC is attempting to use technology to engage people in health, building that technology on empirical data about what works and what does not.

The platform and tools have a clear fit with the goals of HHPC and the populations with which it works. Careful thinking, testing and evaluation research are still needed in order to establish best-practice models for leveraging these emerging technologies and to boost our ability to support health improvement in our community. In conclusion, Kukafka quoted John Dewey, "If the living, experiencing being is an intimate participant in the activities of the world to which it belongs, then knowledge is a mode of participation, valuable in the degree in which it is effective. It cannot be the view of an unconcerned spectator" (Dewey, 1926).

MY HEALTH*e*VET

Kim Nazi, F.A.C.H.E.
Management Analyst, Veterans Health Administration

In response to the Institute of Medicine report, *Crossing the Quality Chasm*, the Veterans Health Administration (VHA) of the Department of Veterans Affairs (VA) began efforts to bring a consumer focus to organization-wide electronic health record development so that patients could directly obtain the benefits of technology. The two major components of eHealth at the VA are the electronic health record—which includes the CPRS (computerized patient record system), BCMA,[6] and VistA imaging,[7] supported by VistA (Veterans Health Information Systems and Technology Architecture)—and the personal health record, My Health*e*Vet. These components offer a number of improvements over the previous system, including more comprehensive records, access to trusted patient education, engagement and action, patient safety, medication reconciliation, patient concordance, wellness reminders, decision support, communication, and patient and provider partnerships.

The development of My Health*e*Vet has been guided by the belief that

---

[6] "Bar Code Medication Administration (BCMA) is a point-of-care software solution that addresses the serious issue of inpatient medication errors by electronically validating and documenting medications for inpatients. It ensures that the patient receives the correct medication in the correct dose, at the correct time, and visually alerts staff when the proper parameters are not met" (Department of Veterans Affairs, 2008a).

[7] The VistA Imaging system makes the complete multimedia patient record available to clinicians and patients (Department of Veterans Affairs, 2008b).

knowledgeable patients are better able to make informed health care decisions, stay healthy, and seek services when they are needed than patients who are not as knowledgeable about their care. In the pilot project now underway, patients are able to access data from the electronic health record, supplement those data with self-entered data, and control access to that information. The pilot project began in 1999 and has about 7,500 participants spread across nine VA Medical Centers. Once the same kinds of features are available in the national My HealtheVet program, the pilot will be discontinued.

In November 2003, on Veterans Day, VA introduced the national My HealtheVet, beginning with some patient education modules. Since then a variety of features have been added, including online prescription refills (which has been one of the most popular features), content centers (oriented to specific conditions or health and wellness), self-assessment tools, health journals and e-logs, veteran-specific conditions, seasonal health reminders, a wellness calendar, and a complete medications view.

My HealtheVet (www.myhealth.va.gov) has three tiers of access. The first tier is intended for visitors, who can view health education libraries and other publicly available content. The second tier is for veterans who self-register for an account and begin to build a personal health record. In particular, patients who register for My HealtheVet can begin to input and track personal information. The third tier of access demands in-person authentication[8] and connects the veteran registration data to the veteran as a VA patient. This authentication allows the veteran access to additional features, such as the ability to view medication names when ordering VA prescription refills and access to the VA medication history as an extract from the VA electronic health record. Many of the screens within My HealtheVet have printer-friendly functions. There is even a printer-friendly wallet card on which patients can choose to print specific data.

There are several different tabs available in My HealtheVet. Using the pharmacy tab, VA patients can refill VA prescriptions, keep track of their prescription history, and even track over-the-counter medications and prescription medications that they are getting from physicians outside the VA. The Research Health tab allows patients to look at multiple media, including interactive images and video on diseases and conditions of interest. There are also direct links to MedLine Plus[9] and Healthwise.[10]

---

[8] Data from the American Customer Satisfaction Index indicate that "in-person authentication" is difficult to understand; therefore, VA will review the language to try to make the information and process understandable to patients in a much more user-friendly way.

[9] MedLine Plus is a website network database of health information provided by the National Library of Medicine and the National Institutes of Health for use by consumers and health care providers.

[10] "Healthwise is a nonprofit organization with a mission to help people make better health decisions. Nearly 100 million times a year, people turn to Healthwise information to

In the Get Care tab, patients can keep track of their providers, their treatment locations and facilities, and health insurance coverage. The Track Health tab allows patients to keep track of their health history, vital signs and readings, test and laboratory results, family health history, military health history, allergies, and immunizations. Patients can also view graphs of self-entered data. Using the printer function they can print these graphs and bring them to a clinic visit. In the pilot program patients are allowed to authorize other persons to have electronic access to their files for a specific amount of time, and this is planned for the national program, as well.

There are nearly 24 million veterans and 259,000 VA staff who are eligible to use the My HealtheVet system. Of the veterans, almost 8 million are enrolled for care in the VA. At this time, there are currently more than 550,000 registered users of My HealtheVet, 71 percent of whom are actually VA patients. As mentioned previously, there is a three-tiered access to the system—visitor, registered members, and authenticated members. There are currently 59,000 veterans who have been in person authenticated and are now able to receive VA prescription medication names as the initial extract from the electronic health record, thereby improving medication reconciliation. More than 5.3 million prescription refills have been processed since August 31, 2005, and more than 16 million visits have been made to the My HealtheVet website since it was launched in November of 2003.

The median age of users of the My HealtheVet is 59, and the age segment with the largest number of users is from 60 to 64 years old. During the past two quarters, however, the greatest population growth occurred in the younger ages—soldiers returning from Iraq and Afghanistan. That population is computer literate and has high expectations for being able to interact via computer with the VA.

VA has implemented the American Customer Satisfaction Index (ACSI) among users of My HealtheVet. Information obtained for that index includes the veteran's period of service, age, and frequency of visits. The majority of users are from the Vietnam War era. Thirty-five percent of users are from 51 to 60 years of age, and 33 percent are from 61 to 70 years. Fifty-one percent of users visit the website approximately once a month, while 25 percent actually visit once a week.

Based on information from the ASCI, the satisfaction with My

---

learn how to do more for themselves, ask for the care they need, and say "no" to the care they don't need. Healthwise partners with health plans, hospitals, disease management companies, and health Web sites to provide up-to-date, evidence-based information to the people they serve. To learn more about the Healthwise Information Therapy (Ix®) Solution, visit www.healthwise.org or call 1.800.706.9646" (Healthwise, 2008).

HealtheVet is high. When asked if they were satisfied with the My HealtheVet program overall, visitors rated My HealtheVet highly, with an average satisfaction rating of 8.3 out of a possible 10. When asked how likely they were to recommend My HealtheVet to someone else, most visitors indicated they would recommend the site with an average likelihood score of 8.6 out of 10. Veterans also indicated that they were highly likely to return to the site and use it, with an average score of 9.1 out of 10.

In addition to providing services through My HealtheVet and assessing consumer satisfaction, the VA is conducting performance evaluations of the reach, effectiveness, adoption, implementation, and maintenance (RE-AIM) of the system. The VA believes that it is important not only to track the effectiveness of an intervention, but also to evaluate the adoption of these tools used by both the patients and the clinicians. The ultimate goal of these evaluations is to learn how to provide access to every veteran in the country in such a way that the system can be maintained over time.

There are many benefits of the My HealtheVet. In terms of health literacy, access to information is a major issue. There is a vast amount of information available to users of the Internet but it is not all necessarily useful or helpful. Access to relevant, trusted, patient health–education tools and resources such as are available at My HealtheVet increases a patient's level of engagement and fosters informed decision making. Ensuring that these sources are highly functional and easy to use, with information presented in a patient-friendly manner is one way that health literacy can be improved. Content development includes input both from experts who pay attention to the language that is used with the goal of making it as understandable as possible, and from the results of focus groups that test the content to make sure patients can understand.

Another benefit to patients is that access to care in multiple settings is facilitated by the VA's electronic health record and My HealtheVet. Such access improves veterans' timely access to services, enhancing utilization management. A veteran could travel to a distant part of the country, for example, and still be able to have a clinician call up a record that stores information from all different sites where the patient has received care. Furthermore, My HealtheVet increases the patients' ability to derive meaning from health information and make informed decisions by combining usable, patient-friendly information in engaging formats with a variety of other tools such as wellness reminders.

My HealtheVet also allows veterans to input information from care provided in community settings. About 40 percent of the VA population receives care outside the VA system so universal secure access to patient health information is critical to providing integrated care coordination among multiple providers.

Finally, personal health records such as those in My Health*e*Vet use technology to facilitate improved communication between patients and health care providers. Secure messaging will add new tools to supplement traditional care interactions. VA is currently in the alpha testing stage of secure messaging.

The contributions of eHealth to the goals of health literacy and improving patient outcomes can be very powerful, Nazi concluded. My Health*e*Vet is transforming health care by enhancing communication and providing veterans access to information that they can understand and use to make good health decisions.

DISCUSSION

George Isham, M.D., M.S.
HealthPartners
Moderator

An audience member asked Kukafka whether the extent to which respondents in the Harlem survey used the Internet for purchasing had any correlation with their level of comfort about obtaining health information. Kukafka responded that while data on commerce was collected, she did not have those data available and was unable to provide an answer.

The same participant, noting that Kukafka's presentation mentioned wariness and mistrust of medical institutions, asked: Do the data indicate that the information would be viewed more credibly if it was derived from the individual's primary care provider or their medical home? If the primary care provider was the author of information on the Internet site, would it be viewed as credible?

That specific question was not asked, Kukafka replied, but the answer to the question is empirical. Currently, however, the data are not yet available to determine the answer. Results of the survey and the focus groups do indicate that the credibility of information from the health provider was rated as very high. On the website, well known community providers serve as creators of content. For example, information is being developed and provided by the Harlem Health Promotion Center and key community health care providers. However, equal time is given to any participant in the community who wishes to contribute. The community itself will then rate the information. If there are blogs provided by a group that forms in the community and there are also blogs created by experts, one could measure hits on the sites in order to evaluate which blogs are used more and thus get a good idea of which contributors are viewed as more credible.

Another audience member said that she is delighted to find that people might doubt all the information provided to them by such sources as a drug company or a physician who might have been detailed by a drug company. What is troubling, she said, is that no one is following the money trail on dietary supplements. For example, individuals read about how they can improve their health by taking Vitamin C, or Vitamin E is marketed in some popular magazine. While there is nothing wrong with marketing these supplements, somehow individuals fail to think about the greed factor with the supplements, which are a multi-billion dollar business. Perhaps one should use individuals' natural skepticism as an educational entrée on things such as dietary supplements which deserve skepticism similar to that directed toward the medical establishment. There is also the issue of the placebo effect which should be part of the educational effort

Those are excellent points, Kukafka responded. The idea is that the website will provide a platform for discourse on such topics. As these things arise, there will be educational opportunities to correct erroneous information. But such information cannot be provided "up front" by the experts because it will then be perceived as not credible. It must be part of the discourse.

Kukafka was asked how large a pool of interactions was needed to have a self-correcting group that arrives at the truth through primary sources as opposed to seeking out experts. She responded that it is not known what the necessary number is. The available data show that whatever the size of the population using a wiki, only a small number of individuals in that population will actually make edits. One has to be able to divide the population into those who are making corrections and those who are only viewing. It is interesting that if one examines the numbers of hits for wiki sites versus those sites based on health expert design, the wiki sites tend to draw larger numbers.

Another audience member said that wikis are being used to evaluate various professionals. For example, in San Francisco a website was established recently to evaluate police officers, but it was immediately taken down. Perhaps there are aspects of wikis that could be used to evaluate one's health care providers in terms of their sensitivity or competency in health literacy.

Yet another audience member said that she was concerned that, with the use of wikis, someone might actually act on health information before it is corrected.

Kukafka was asked how liability is being addressed. She responded that there is a disclaimer on the site and that editorial control group will be monitoring the content. Asked about how content development for non-English-speaking populations was proceeding, Kukafka responded that currently the portal is being developed in English because of the complexity involved. There is a complementary project that will link the portal to a more traditional personal health record that has the traditional functions such as patient reminders and prescription refills. There will also be point-of-care patient education.

The portal, however, provides very different kinds of content—in particular, more actionable content. When a doctor tells a patient to control his or her blood pressure, for example, the "how to do it" is the part that is often missing and, furthermore, is very community-specific. The portal is a place to go to hear about what others have tried to do, what they have done or could not do, as well as a place to join groups or start groups aimed at accomplishing specific things.

One participant commented that the statistics provided on the number of people who have access to and use the Internet are encouraging. She then asked Kukafka if, when conducting the telephone survey, the interviewers probed those individuals who do not have a computer or did not use the Internet in order to determine what the barriers to use were? And, if so, will the project begin to address some of those issues? Kukafka responded that the interviewers did probe and that some of the information on barriers was presented. Fear of pornography and fraud was actually of higher importance than being able to understand the information. Will the project be able to do something about all the barriers? The answer is no. What the project can do is encourage discourse among the participants during which the barriers might emerge and can then be discussed.

In terms of such barriers as having to wait in long lines at the library to use the computer or having only limited hours when the library is open, the hope is that the community will begin to build capacity in order to reduce some of those barriers. One of the most interesting comments about the portal was "This is not a website, it's an action, it is activism." The portal can assist a ground-up effort and provide the platform for discourse and activism out of which change will occur.

On the subject of the Harlem community, a participant said that there are a variety of factors that are not directly addressed by eHealth, such as the social determinants of health, including lower education and lower employment. It seems that people are thinking that eHealth will provide a panacea to bridge the gap in health disparities. But how likely is it that that will really happen? Isn't it necessary to address the broader social determinants of health and not depend on eHealth bridging the gap?

Kukafka responded that empirical evidence will be necessary to determine the degree to which the Harlem approach is successful. It is likely that there will be early adopters, as in the diffusion of any technology, but there will be people who have significantly more barriers to adoption, and it is doubtful that 100 percent of the population will be reached.

One participant said that while the approaches taken by the VA and Harlem are different, they are related, and it is important to determine which outcomes are desired by the different systems. It appears that VA is looking at the more traditional outcomes such as utilization of services. What outcomes is the Harlem project looking for?

Kukafka responded that the HHPC project is conducting a cohort study with the entire user base to look at such things as changes in attitudes, beliefs, the way the site is used, the extent to which different functions of the system are used, and if the experts are being downloaded or used more than the community generated material. Whether or not the outcomes can be examined depends on funding.

In response, the same questioner said that it appears that HHPC has recognized culture, language, and trust as large barriers and is attempting to design a system to inform users and so address those barriers. That is incredibly important, but it also raises such questions as whether it would be better to have a large number of people who engage in discussions about flu shots or to have a higher rate of flu vaccination. How can one handle such issues? Kukafka responded that it is hoped that if there is a great deal of discourse around flu vaccination, then flu vaccinations would increase. If that does not happen, however, then it will be important to examine the discourse in detail, in order to determine what it was about and why it did not lead to increased vaccinations. Ultimately, the HHPC project is looking for both process and outcome measures. Understanding the process better should identify issues and barriers where new interventions need to be developed, which would then, one hopes, lead to improved outcomes.

One participant said that he was intrigued by the juxtaposition of two approaches—one related to the Harlem project and the other related to the VA. A great deal of research has demonstrated that the VA is incredibly effective in eliminating or reducing health disparities and their approach is very innovative, despite the fact that their population is elderly and has, perhaps, low literacy. What is the VA doing that makes it so effective, that results in it getting 15,000 hits a day?

Nazi responded that the VA has taken a very comprehensive strategy—not just enacting technology, but also implementing technology in a way that reaches people where they are. Knowing that veterans may not have access to a computer, the VA made sure that computers were placed in every medical center for use by veterans. Data show that while veterans access their personal health record they are also accessing the health education libraries. The most downloaded document on the site is a PDF called 5 Steps For Safer Health Care.

Offering value also means offering such programs as online prescription refills, which was of more importance to veterans than any other option. The ACSI data show that the most desired options for online service now are appointment view followed by appointment scheduling. In response, with the secure messaging initiative, VA is building templates to make it very easy for patients to request appointments online. Other services of importance are the ability to engage in secure messaging and the ability to communicate electronically with patients' clinicians.

Because veterans know about the pilot project, it is important for VA to move quickly to make these features available in the national program. While the technology is fairly easy, it takes time to build the business process and the organizational framework at all the sites. For that reason, VA has taken an incremental approach aimed at ensuring that each step is done correctly before moving to the next service.

One participant asked if those who enrolled in the VA Track Health had better health outcomes on average than the members of the VA population who did not enroll. Nazi responded that this is an important research question. Because VA has a research branch, those involved in informatics at VA are pressing for a collaborative effort with VA researchers to study such questions as: Do personal health records make a difference? Do users have better health outcomes? Are they more highly satisfied?

Some research questions are quite complex, such as looking at clinical outcomes over time, but there is a great deal of interest in pursuing questions about eHealth. VA is poised to create a research summit to help develop policy frameworks for how research is to be carried out. The personal health record is a new frontier and requires a multidisciplinary stakeholder approach to make sure the infrastructure is in place to support the research.

One audience member noted that Nazi said the VA would like, ultimately, to give patients access to progress notes and clinical information. Is that information going to be transformed in a way that makes it easily understandable? When one thinks about medical progress notes and how cryptic they might be, will there be an intermediate step to translate the information into something more useful to patients?

Nazi responded that, in the pilot, there has been a narrow focus on answering whether this could be done in a secure way, and if it is done, will patients find it to be of value. From the pilot responses, the answer is yes, although one particular piece that translated clinical reminders into patient-friendly wellness reminders appears to be most easily understood by patients. In terms of the broader question, one of the advantages of building the system incrementally is that one can spend time focused on the different pieces. At present, VA is conducting a field test of offering laboratory test results in order to obtain feedback on the system. In some cases it is not possible to change the readability of the material.

One approach in such situations might be to supplement the data with materials that enrich and support patients' understanding, for example by providing places to obtain additional information and resources to help patients make decisions.

Another approach that VA has worked on in response to an executive order is to offer quality information about delivery of services. Rather than just put forth a report card about quality metrics for a particular facility, clinic, or physician, VA opted to integrate the sharing of quality information into My HealtheVet.

The longer-term goal is to move from generalized reports about the quality of a facility to provider-specific reports, which are then translated into something of value to the patient, such as, Is my blood pressure under control? Is my blood sugar controlled?

An audience member suggested that as one gains more information about one's own personal health record, there may be things in the record that one did not hear when visiting the clinician. Will the VA have a mechanism to allow patients to type questions back to their clinicians for clarification, or is there another way to obtain clarification? Nazi responded that one of the things that emerged from the pilot was that it is very important to patients that the content of their medical record be correct. When that information is released, there must be an easy way for patients to identify things that may need to be corrected. Soon, with one click, a patient will be able to send a secure message to a triage group which then sends it on to the best person to handle the message. The idea that patients should be able to relay information or questions is very interesting and something worth thinking about.

4

Outcomes and Challenges of eHealth Approaches: Panel 2

USING TECHNOLOGY TO IMPROVE
MIGRANT HEALTH CARE DELIVERY

Cynthia Solomon
Chief Executive Officer, Access Strategies, Inc.

MiVIA is a patient electronic personal health record (PHR) originally designed to engage a very vulnerable population—migrant and seasonal farm workers—in their own health care through the use of a personal health record. It was later expanded to include other vulnerable populations such as the homeless, those with special needs, women, and children. The MiVIA project is a collaborative effort of St. Joseph Health System in Sonoma County, California; the Community Health Resource Development Center; and Vineyard Workers Services.

In 2002 and 2003 developers of the new system held meetings with farm workers and settled agricultural workers to explain the concept of the PHR and to ask them what information they would want to carry with them and have accessible to them. The developers quickly learned, for instance, that the participants did not want to be called users or patients or consumers; they wished to be called members. The members named the system MiVIA, which means "my way" in Spanish.

MiVIA has evolved over the years. In 2003 it was a consumer portal for information storage on migrant and farm worker members. By 2005 it included a clinician portal that offered clinicians access to the personal health record (with member permission), but the data entered were read-only. By 2005 MiVIA had expanded to include members of the homeless community. In 2007 four hospitals were using it as an electronic medical record and it had expanded its member rolls to include special needs children.

The resulting PHR, which was designed with input from the members, is Web-based, and compliant with HIPAA (the Health Insurance Portability and Accountability Act). It is now being licensed to hospitals and clinics for use with mobile populations. Additionally, it serves as an affordable electronic health record for small clinics.

When the MiVIA pilot project started in 2003, it had a goal of enrolling 50 migrant workers. That figure quickly became 250, then 300, then 400. Because MiVIA serves a very mobile population of migrant workers who may access many different clinics and health care systems from San Diego all the way up the coast to Alaska, it serves as a bridge among these health systems. It promotes continuity of care and engages and empowers members as active partners in their own health care.

MiVIA stores medical and dental information and provides a photo identification and emergency information card which includes the member's name, health conditions, the last provider seen, any allergies, and other special information, such as presence of implanted medical devices. MiVIA also includes an e-mail account offering a "permanent" address and provides information and resources with links to other health information resources, primarily to MedLine Plus, but also to some other health websites. Both family and individual memberships are available.

It is interesting to note that 7 out of 10 of the providers engaged in MiVIA had not heard about MedLine Plus before getting involved with MiVIA. Once they learn about it, however, they love it. And it is not only providers who appreciate having the additional information available from MedLine Plus, but members appreciate it as well. One story illustrates the value of this resource. About a year and a half ago, an older gentleman came to the resource center with his daughter. The gentlemen was supposed to take seven medications but the daughter told an outreach worker that, while her father needed the medications, he did not take them. The outreach worker and the daughter sat with the father, logged on to MedLine Plus, looked up every medication, and printed the information in Spanish. That was what was needed to engage the gentleman in his health care so that he took his medication. The small amount of effort required to log into MedLine Plus and retrieve information from it made all the difference in that patient's care.

MiVIA has a clinician portal for professional entry and verification. A clinician can go to www.mivia.org, sign up as a clinician, and run a test account to check out the system. The log-in is also available in Spanish, although it is somewhat more limited. There are approximately 5,000

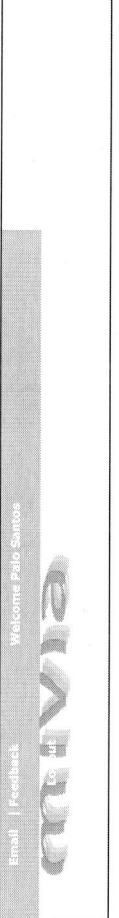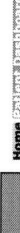

FIGURE 4-1 Patient dashboard.
SOURCE: Solomon, 2008.

MiVIA members in Sonoma County and about 1,100 of them use the Spanish version.

One useful feature of the system is the patient dashboard (see Figure 4-1). On the dashboard the member's information is on the left-hand side. Among other things it tracks medications and providers, and it provides all the information needed to fill out the forms on a physician visit.

The member identification card is probably one of the most popular features of MiVIA. The card can be printed anytime. If a change is made to the PHR (e.g., adding a medication), the card is reprinted and the new information appears. If a member who does not speak English visits a clinic or hospital where no translator is available, this card can be used to provide pertinent information and access to the patient's PHR.

MiVIA has many features. It is a single database with both member access and clinician access. A member can grant a clinician access to his or her MiVIA record. There is also "on-the-fly" clinician sign up, meaning that if a clinician wants a MiVIA member to see a specialist, the member can give the specialist immediate permission to access his or her record. There is also a Spanish version which is experiencing some challenges that will be described later. There is a service wheel which identifies resources by special population or region. Resources include information about employment, transportation, housing, community services, health services, and legal assistance. So, for example, if a member is in San Diego but is going to Sonoma to work for a while, he or she can click on housing and locate the different services available to him for migrant housing.

The most recent version of MiVIA includes a feature that allows a continuity-of-care record (CCR) to be downloaded into a computer or another electronic medical record system. MiVIA is currently working with two electronic medical record companies to test this feature. MiVIA also has a complete audit-and-edit trail with date and time stamping. The system is located in a collocation facility that has managed servers. Encryption, SSL,[1] and secure log-in and passwords are used.

Member suggestions have led to a number of enhancements to the system. The success of MiVIA is due primarily to the outreach and lay outreach workers, or *promotores*. They are the champions of MiVIA. They conduct the enrollment and provide the training in the use of MiVIA. They also provide cultural and social support and check in with the members about their use of MiVIA.

The *promotores* are provided with a training and enrollment manual that is very simple to use. There are about three training sessions each year that the *promotores* can attend. Each session lasts about two and a half hours and starts with the basics—what the computer is used for and how

---

[1] SSL stands for secure sockets layer which is a technology used to protect websites.

to access different programs. There is a quick overview of the Internet, with a brief look at different sites, and the session also covers the purpose of MiVIA, its use, and how to enter and access data. Since the training can be intense, *promotores* often return for a repeat session.

When MiVIA first began, most of those who enrolled did not have an e-mail account, so MiVIA provided an e-mail account for anyone who needed one. Within a few years that changed so that most of those enrolling today come in to the system with their own e-mail accounts, indicating awareness of the Internet.

Similar to the patient dashboard described earlier, there is also a clinician dashboard that MiVIA makes available to health care providers. Using this dashboard, a MiVIA clinician can, with a member's permission, use the member's log-in, password, or limited-access code to enroll the member on the clinician's list of patients. This enables the clinician to pull up patient data.

The clinician portal features an alphabetical list of individual clinicians or clinics, and patient lists by organization. Access to patient records is with the owner's permission only. With that permission, clinicians can access patient records online at any time and from any place. Data entry is protected, as it is read-only to members and other clinicians.

The latest version of MiVIA uses the SOAP[2] format for data entry. This version allows providers to record whether the nature of a patient visit is preventive, emergency, or chronic care. The version also has a telemedicine component which becomes the record between the patient, the specialist, and the provider. Those granted access can retrieve a summary medical report that can be downloaded or else can go to specific parts of the record detailing such things as immunizations, medical office visits, and allergies. The information can also be shared across platforms.

There are many member benefits of MiVIA. It reduces the divide between those who have access to digital and information technology and those who do not. It facilitates access to health and community services, clinics, and libraries. The *promotores*, when teaching about MiVIA, teach farm workers and their families to use the local library, taking them to the library, showing them around, and showing them how to access the Internet. Because the members have MiVIA cards, they are able to get library cards, which they were not eligible for before. Members become more engaged in their community. MiVIA also promotes health care literacy and peace of mind. Members know their information is safely stored and can follow them wherever they go for services.

MiVIA has applications for children with special needs who have

---

[2] SOAP stands for subjective, objective, assessment plan. The SOAP format is used to document observations and care provided.

multiple conditions as well as for the homeless. In the case of the children, MiVIA eases the burden of parents who are busy with multiple medical appointments, providing an easy way to carry health information with them at all times. In the case of the homeless, clients have a concise document on which to store health information. Relevant personal data from the U.S. Department of Housing and Urban Development can be copied and pasted into MiVIA. The MiVIA photo ID allows clients to pick up their prescription voucher at local pharmacies.

In Fall 2007, the St. Joseph Health System conducted a telephone member satisfaction follow-up survey. Of 613 members, 40 percent of the people enrolled said that they log on to MiVIA on a regular basis. Eight percent (50) members had no prior computer experience and received basic computer training from MiVIA. Eighty-seven percent of members enrolled did not have a computer in their home.

MiVIA also has a disease-management tool. The first disease targeted was diabetes, and work has now begun on asthma. With the diabetes-management tool, members can track their blood sugar and weight, graphing this information and sharing it with their health care providers. MiVIA is also working with several regional health information organizations (RHIOs) and EMR linkages.

MiVIA is currently working in Sonoma County, California, with mobile medical and dental clinics, community clinics, a family practice residency "bridge" clinic for diabetics, a homeless center, and a resource center. MiVIA also works with two hospitals and three rural clinics in the California Central Valley. In Hood River, Oregon, MiVIA is working with a hospital, a mobile medical clinic, and a rural clinic. In the Finger Lakes region of New York MiVIA is working with five clinics, three voucher sites,[3] and an integrated network and is involved in telemedicine. Hospitals that join MiVIA use it as a method for health information exchange between local physicians' offices, their patients, and the hospital.

Several lessons have been learned since MiVIA began in 2003. First, each community is different. Second, the value of the photo ID cannot be overstated. Third, *promotores* are invaluable resources trusted by members. Fourth, members gain computer skills through the use of MiVIA. Finally, it is extremely valuable to partner with local libraries and community-based organizations to provide computers and classes in English as a second language.

One of the challenges MiVIA faces in serving limited-English-

---

[3] A voucher is an agreement between a provider and the voucher program (usually a migrant health grantee), to reimburse a provider, who is usually in a distant location, for health services provided to the migrant worker. Voucher sites are local providers who are contracted with on a per-visit basis.

proficiency (LEP) members is that printed and online content is not easily available in Spanish, with the exception of MedLine Plus, and appropriate translation services are difficult to locate. MiVIA's first translation effort was carried out by a university and cost a substantial amount of money, which was paid for by a grant. Two years later MiVIA learned that it was not an appropriate translation. It was a word-for-word translation and, as such, did not make sense. MiVIA has received a great deal of criticism about that translation and is in the process of trying to identify the correct technical and financial resources to remedy the error. Still, despite its problems, the Spanish translation is being used for now since there is, as yet, nothing better.

A final challenge relates to quality. Those who work in the field of electronic health records and information exchange are so involved with issues of technology, privacy, security, getting the project out, and preparing for interoperability that that they have not yet put in place a mechanism to measure the quality and content of the translation. This is a key challenge.

Solomon made several recommendations for future efforts to construct patient-centered health information technology. First, when issuing requests for proposals, it should be a prerequisite for funding that the proposal should include provisions for serving LEP individuals. Second, resources should be made available to assist organizations in accessing, measuring, and deploying health content that is relevant and respectful of cultural differences. Finally, because many individuals in vulnerable populations do not read or do not read well, the development of downloadable audio and video content should be encouraged.

Although many talk about the huge investment of resources needed to develop health information technology, the total amount of funding for MiVIA through the 6 years of its development is less than $600,000. This is not a huge investment, considering the benefits that accrue.

Solomon concluded with a vision for the future of MiVIA and other personal health records. In that vision, these tools make it possible for both physician and patient information to be sent directly to the PHR from any electronic health record; there are condition-specific modules for self management; access to critical information is available 24 hours a day, 7 days a week; and the tools have the ability to bridge language barriers between patients and providers.

A USER-CENTERED PERSONAL HEALTH RECORD: THE DESIGN AND DEVELOPMENT OF THE SHARED CARE PLAN

Dawn Gauthier, M.I.S.
Web Usability Designer, PeaceHealth

In 2001 the Robert Wood Johnson Foundation awarded a Pursuing Perfection grant to Whatcom County, Washington (the only community to receive such a grant) to implement a chronic disease model, including the development of a user-centered personal health record (PHR). The project was also supported by a patient safety grant from the Agency for Healthcare Research and Quality. With the publication of *Crossing the Quality Chasm* (IOM, 2001), those working on the project kept in mind the report's six aims for improvement[4] and the ten rules[5] for the health care system as design work proceeded.

Whatcom County had been very much interested in designing a patient-centered health care system. Development of a user-centered electronic health record, the Shared Care Plan, fit well with the activities of the County. The project began with a focus on chronic conditions and the design of a chronic-disease-management tool. The involvement of patients pushed the design in the direction of a personal health record.

The design goals of the Shared Care Plan, which was an endeavor of the entire community including all the providers, were to

- facilitate patients' interactions with the health care system, supporting the virtual Care Team concept, and planned care, and to ensure the "nothing about me without me" perspective of the patient;
- offer patients a tool that fosters a sense of responsibility for their own health and encourages them to learn about and practice principles of self-management (such as maintaining a medication list), thereby encouraging educated and engaged patients;
- provide a tool that enables patients to feel safer because they are informed and in control; and

---

[4] The six aims for improvement for the health care system are that the system must be safe, effective, patient-centered, timely, efficient, and equitable (IOM, 2001).

[5] The 10 rules for the health care system are that care should be based on continuous healing relationships, there should be customization based on patient needs and values, the patient should be the source of control, there should be shared knowledge and the free flow of information, there should be evidence-based decision making, safety should be a system property, there is a need for transparency, the health system should anticipate patient needs, there should be a continuous decrease in waste, and there should be cooperation among clinicians (IOM, 2001).

- give patients access to their clinical information from multiple community health care systems so that they may organize it into a single meaningful lifelong personal health record and then make appropriate parts of that record available to those who need it at the patient-owner's discretion.

The second goal may be of particular interest to those attending this workshop because of its health literacy aspects. The idea behind the goal is that if patients could be encouraged to use the Shared Care Plan, even if they did not understand everything they encountered, not only would their health literacy increase but, if their Shared Care Plan was up to date, they would be in a good position to deal with any issues that might arise in their health care.

There are currently more than 1,400 Shared Care plans in Whatcom County. There are also a couple of pilot sites in Oregon. The regions in which the plans are being implemented are the PeaceHealth regions.

Patient involvement was key to development. The user-centered design approach is more than just a methodology; it is a philosophy and a process in which the tasks, needs, wants and limitations of the end user of a system (in this case, the patients) are given extensive attention at each stage of the design process.

Jakob Nielsen (2005) developed the following key end-user principles or "rights" for user-centered design. First, people should be considered superior to technology. While that may seem obvious, there are those involved in technology development and programming who may sometimes need to be reminded of this. Second is the right to empowerment. Third, users have the right to simplicity, that is, to have things that are well-designed, easy to use, and designed to complete the task one needs to complete, not someone else's idea of what one needs to complete. Finally, people have the right to have their time respected. One can waste a great deal of time using poorly designed technology. Such technology is very frustrating and can be intimidating.

Through an approach called user research, system designers working on the Shared Care Plan project set out to determine what tasks patients were actually attempting to accomplish. They observed, they listened to patients tell their stories, and they asked questions about why patients did things in a certain way. Several approaches were used to gather information including one-on-one contextual interviews, usability testing of design ideas and prototypes, patient focus groups, and surveys.

A very popular approach is the use of focus groups. It is important in such groups to make sure you have a range of representation including

- patients who most successfully navigate the health care system;

- patients who are healthy and rarely use the system;
- patients who fully understand what you are trying to do (may be health care professionals themselves); and
- patients who have no idea what you are trying to do.

The difficulty with the focus group approach is that one can end up with "group-think." That is, people begin agreeing with each other even if what they hear is not actually how they do things. Furthermore, people may say that they do things in a particular way but when they are actually observed, they are doing it differently.

In user-centered design one figures out what patients are trying to do, designs something that one thinks will allow patients to accomplish their tasks, tests the design with the patients, and then evaluates whether the design worked or not. The resulting feedback is then used to refine the system design as necessary. One does not need a fully functioning prototype to evaluate a design; one can use ideas and drawings on paper for the tests.

The best approach is probably one-on-one contextual design. In this approach one goes into the field to talk with patients. During such interviews one might accompany patients to physician office visits and watch their interactions with physicians. One might even, accompanied by the patient, look through the patient's medicine cabinet.

An important part of user-centered design is producing a task analysis, because such an analysis crystallizes the design work. In a task analysis one lists all the tasks that are observed and then prioritizes the tasks based on how important each task is to the patients. This helps define the scope and focus of the product.

In terms of scope, for example, even though survey after survey has shown that the thing patients most want to be able to do is refill their medications online, and even though project designers knew it was a high priority for patients, the decision was made to not include that in the personal health record. That decision was made because the task was too large to accomplish for every single health organization in the community, and the Shared Health Plan is a community-wide resource. It was an intentional decision, therefore, to leave that tool out of the scope of the PHR product.

Task analysis also serves to keep design and development work focused on the task at hand. It is easy to get off track because there are so many interesting and wonderful features that can be tried in this arena. A task analysis, however, focuses designers on what patients are trying to accomplish. This focus clears a great deal of static from the design process.

Most importantly, when one has user research and a task analysis in hand, decisions are made by referencing user data rather than relying on opinions and assumptions. This is very important, especially if one is working with health care professionals. Such professionals frequently believe that they know what is best for patients and that, if patients would just do things the way the professionals say, everything will work out fine. So user research is a way to keep the focus on the patients. When this was done, it was found that patients' tools are very different from the tools one might build for clinicians and health care professionals.

Finally, the design work focused on how to support the tasks that were identified, rather than making up the tasks that one thinks patients should be doing.

The project also had a Patient Action and Advisory Committee. Gauthier strongly recommended that anyone designing technology for patients convene such a group. It makes it easier to find patients to work with, and the committee members invigorate staff, keeping them focused on the reasons the product is being developed.

Much of the design work and problem solving for the system was tested with patients using a wireframe[6] before a single line of code was written. Patients were given a graphic representation of a Web page and told they could use their finger as a mouse to click on the various options. They were then asked questions such as, "What would you click on to add a new medication?" Using a wireframe with patients allows the designer to determine where changes should be made. It also allows for rapid iterations that bring one closer and closer to a really great design that most patients will be able to pick up and use quite easily.

The following examples illustrate how a task was designed in the user interface. The first task was for a patient to be able to find the generic name of a medication. There is a great deal of confusion among patients over the myriad names for a single drug. The design decision was made to always pair the brand name with the generic name so that patients always see the two together (see Figure 4-2). When patients add medications to their lists, the lists will always show both the brands and, when available, the generic pairing. The page also shows the patient which strengths of the medication are available, a piece of information that patients were very interested in knowing.

---

[6] A wireframe "is a visualization tool for presenting proposed functions, structure and content of a Web page or Web site. A wireframe separates the graphic elements of a Web site from the functional elements in such a way that Web teams can easily explain how users will interact with the Web site. A typical wireframe includes (1) key page elements and their location, such as header, footer, navigation, content objects, branding elements, (2) grouping of elements, such as side bars, navigation bars, content areas, (3) labeling, page title, navigation links, headings to content objects, and (4) place holders, content text and images" (Jupitermedia Corporation, 2008).

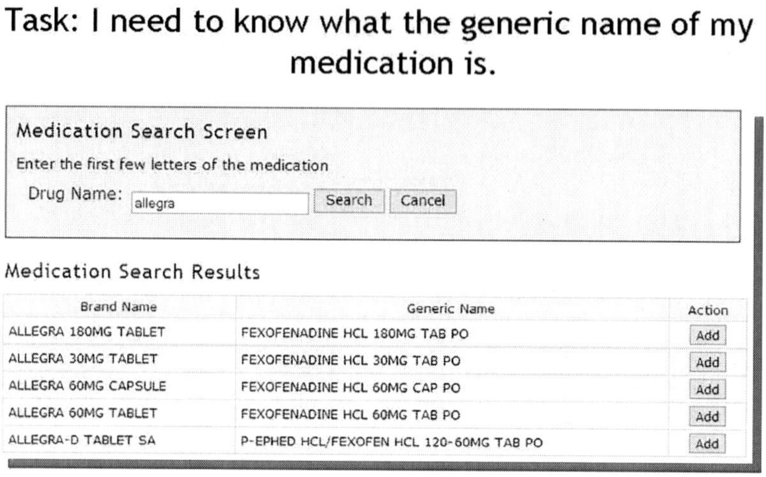

Task: I need to know what the generic name of my medication is.

Medication Search Screen		
Enter the first few letters of the medication		
Drug Name: allegra	Search	Cancel

Medication Search Results

Brand Name	Generic Name	Action
ALLEGRA 180MG TABLET	FEXOFENADINE HCL 180MG TAB PO	Add
ALLEGRA 30MG TABLET	FEXOFENADINE HCL 30MG TAB PO	Add
ALLEGRA 60MG CAPSULE	FEXOFENADINE HCL 60MG CAP PO	Add
ALLEGRA 60MG TABLET	FEXOFENADINE HCL 60MG TAB PO	Add
ALLEGRA-D TABLET SA	P-EPHED HCL/FEXOFEN HCL 120-60MG TAB PO	Add

FIGURE 4-2 Task.
SOURCE: Gauthier, 2008.

Another task was to allow the patient to find the name of a medication he or she took in the past because it was effective and he or she would like to take it again. Amazingly, many patient records and medication lists are structured so that only active medications are shown. Yet there are a number of valid and legitimate reasons that patients might need to access their discontinued medication lists, so the project designed a discontinued-medication section in the Shared Care Plan. The system is designed so that it does not require the patient to do any work to maintain the list. The patient simply takes a medication off the active-medication list and, unless the patient states that the removal was entered in error, the medication will automatically be put onto the patient's discontinued medication list.

Another task that patients are often faced with is to quickly communicate their health information to a new doctor. As in the case of MiVIA discussed earlier, the wallet-sized card provided with the Shared Care Plan is valued by both patients and their health care professionals. The card provides a concise summary of some of the most pertinent information in the personal health record and can be easily printed. If one were to print the entire Shared Care Plan, by contrast, it could be 15 to 20 pages long.

Since one of the goals of the Shared Care Plan is to enable patients to communicate with their health care professionals, and because health care professionals were logging into the system, it became necessary to support clinician tasks in addition to patient tasks. For example, a clinician seeing a patient for the first time who finds no allergies listed on the plan may want to know if the patient really has no allergies or if the patient has just not yet filled out that section of the Shared Care Plan. It often takes patients several sittings to fill out the entire plan which means that there will often be varying levels of completion. The design has to allow patients to check a box that explicitly states that the patient has no known allergies so that the answer is not ambiguous to the clinicians.

There were numerous challenges encountered in designing the system. One set of challenges related to privacy and security. How, for example, can one design the system to safely provide patients access to their private health care information over the Internet, yet still allow needed information to be shared in an emergency situation? Other issues in this area included how clinicians would log in and how usage would be audited.

The Shared Care Plan was designed so patients can explicitly give view-only or fully-edit access to their care team members (see Figure 4-3). In Whatcom County about 99 percent of the physicians participate in the local health care network which means that patients can easily look up their various local health care providers and add them to their care teams. Patients can invite family members and friends to be part of their care team as well by using the invitation mechanism. Patients are the ones who determine who is on their care team.

Providing appropriate emergency access was another issue in the area of privacy and security. In the situation illustrated in Figure 4-3, access is given to a group called Community Clinicians. This is a way to group all the community clinicians together whom the patient has not explicitly listed on the care team. By granting community clinicians access to the records, the patient is saying that anyone who needs to access the Shared Care Plan in an emergency may have access. Alternatively, patients can also block access to anyone who is not explicitly listed on the care team.

Figure 4-4 illustrates the privacy flag feature. In this example, a patient is adding a new diagnosis (sleep apnea) to the diagnosis list. At the bottom of every record that the patient adds to the Shared Care Plan, there is the privacy flag indicated by a padlock icon. When the patient checks the box by the padlock, the team list is displayed at the bottom of the page and the patient decides who will be able to access that diagnosis. This was a feature that patients requested. Patients did not want a blanket yes/no setting for access to a record for the entire care team; they wanted instead to decide which individuals on the care team would have access.

The system also produces a summary of who has accessed the record, the health care facility and department of those who accessed the record, and the date on which the access occurred. Patients can view that summary access screen at any time. If the patient sees something

Care Team Members (HELP)

Care Team Members are people and/or organizations who help you manage your health. Anyone who you feel has a role in your health care can be part of your Care Team.

Sort | Add New

Appts.	Name	Contact	Role/Description	Access Level	Comments	Action
	Dawn Gauthier	360-756-0219	Patient	Admin: Fully Edit		Edit
	Community Clinicians		Emergencies & Treatment	Fully Edit	Click [Edit] to adjust clinical access to your Shared Care Plan.	Edit
10/11/2007	Erin Baumgart	360-555-5050 ebaum@email.com	Gynecologist	Fully Edit		Edit
10/4/2007	Lilly Longview	666-444-4444 ll@emai.com	Primary Care Physician	View Only		Edit
7/1999; 9/2000; 11/2004	Lulu Fritzenbacher	(360) 756-0219 lbach@allergist.com	Allergist	Fully Edit		Edit
	Marcia Brady	1234567890 mbrady@email.com	Family Member	View Only		Edit

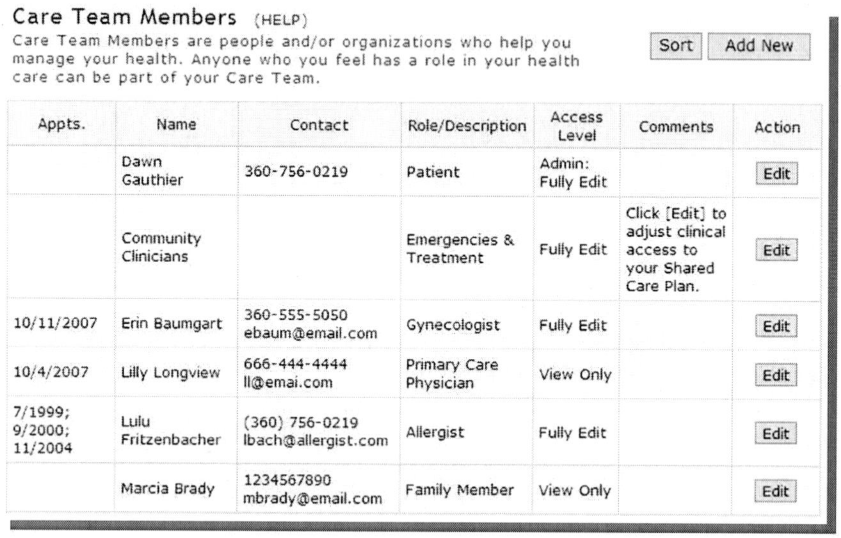

FIGURE 4-3 Care team members.
SOURCE: Gauthier, 2008.

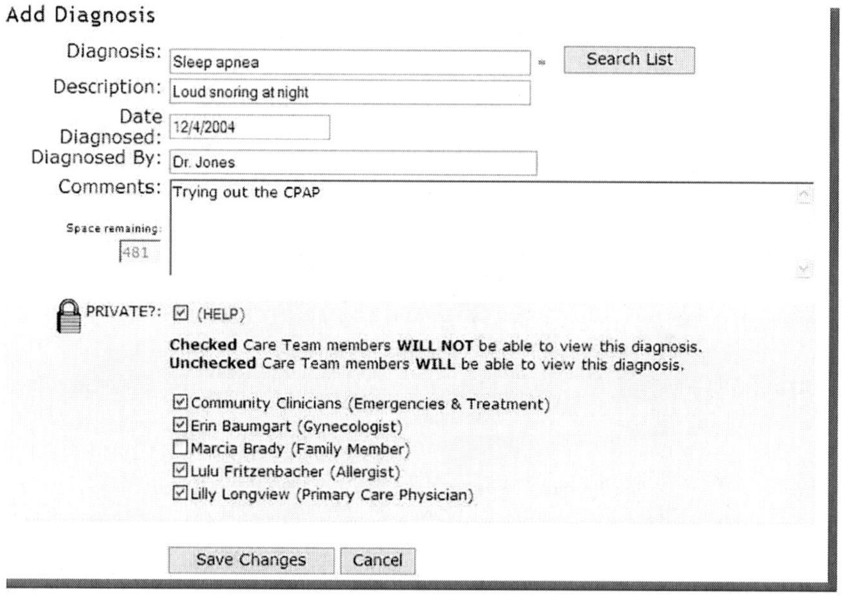

FIGURE 4-4 Add diagnosis.
SOURCE: Gauthier, 2008.

troubling, he or she can call the Shared Care Plan office and ask the staff there to look into the situation. Shared Care Plan staff can also audit the entire database, which is not available through user interface. If a patient alerts staff to a problem because a name appears on the audit trail that the patient does not recognize, staff can go into the database and re-create what happened. No editing activity is ever deleted.

Although there are some nice front-end privacy controls in the Shared Care Plan, there is not, as yet, a policy that discloses who has access to the back end of a PHR; is it 5 people or 100 people? With a definite policy in place that discloses this type of information, patients would be better able to make determinations about how secure the back end of a PHR system is.

In addition to challenges surrounding privacy and security, there have also been challenges involving health literacy. There is a great deal of accumulated wisdom available from patients who have navigated the health care system. The features and functionalities of the Shared Care Plan were designed based on the tasks that engaged patients are performing. But how does one explain these features and functions to someone who is interacting with the health care system for the first time? The concepts in, for example, managing a medication list are extremely complex. Designers spent a great deal of time on the medication list because there were a large number of things that patients needed to understand and to do, but there is a real problem in preparing new participants to comprehend these concepts.

The Shared Care Plan was developed specifically for a chronic-disease population. Once it was turned into a more general personal health record the target audience expanded and the need for meeting patients at their own knowledge level increased. One thing that has been done to mitigate the problem is giving patients the choice to deactivate sections in the Shared Care Plan that they find they are not using. For example, there is a goal-setting/next steps section that chronic-disease patients find very useful but that someone who is healthy and just wants to have a record may not need to use.

The platform approach may be one way of managing this problem. With HealthVault, Microsoft is constructing a basic platform that allows people to build tools that can then be plugged into the platform. This avoids the problem of each group having to do all the work of designing and building the functions of the platform over and over again. In the future, it is likely that there will be a greater variety of tools which serve many different audiences and which can be built more quickly and then plugged into HealthVault.

Many individuals have never heard of a personal health record. To educate potential users, drop-in labs were organized that allowed people to sit with an expert who provided hands-on attention while the users worked through the system. To build awareness, presentations were given at such locations as community centers, senior centers, and churches. Once a few people became excited about the Shared Care Plan they acted as ambassadors, talking with friends and family, and spreading the idea. This was a very successful way of spreading ideas and getting people to sign up.

The final challenge is management of patient expectations. This is incredibly difficult. It takes a great deal of explaining to get people to sign up for the personal health record. Once they sign up, they are very pleased to find they can add any of their clinicians in the community to their care team and set the access level for each person. But once they have done this, they tend to expect that the clinicians will be constantly logging on to the PHR to record and access information. Not all clinicians, however, entirely engage in using the system.

Patients also expected to be able to log in to the system and immediately have all of their health care records electronically available for them to download into their personal health record. But as Marchibroda mentioned, only a small percentage of physicians use electronic health records. Thus, it was necessary to work with patients to explain the limitations and to temper their expectations.

Another common patient expectation was that a critical mass of clinicians would be engaged. It is a great deal of work to fill out the Shared Care Plan and it is even more work to maintain it. Patients were lucky if one of their clinicians was a participant in the Pursuing Perfection Project. A large number of patients did not have any officially participating clinicians which meant they did not see their clinicians participating. Unfortunately there were a number of stories of patients taking their printed Share Care Plan to a clinician visit, even the wallet-size version, only to have the clinician completely disregard it, even throw it into the trash can in one extreme case. Imagine the effect that had on the patient's perception of the value of filling out the large amount of information in the Shared Care Plan.

Patients will understand the value of PHRs only when they start actually seeing them significantly improving their experiences within the health care system. (e.g., not repeating their medication lists verbally, not having to fill out repetitive forms, etc.). In other words, patients won't value PHRs until their own clinicians value and use them.

Recently, emergency medical services (EMS) in Whatcom County have decided to participate with the system. Ambulances have installed wireless Internet, and now EMS has the ability, when receiving a 911 call, to cross-walk the telephone number with a patient's Shared Care Plan, if there is one. If the patient has given the community clinicians ability to access the PHR, the ambulance drivers can actually look up information as they are driving to the patient's house. This is very appealing to patients.

Improvements to the system are always being made. A new version of the Shared Care Plan was recently launched, for example. While it appears similar to users, there is a great deal of new technology in place, including new support for localization (such as language). This version is being piloted in New Zealand and Sweden, among other places. There is also a beta version that will enable integration with emerging platforms such as Microsoft's HealthVault.

The original version of the Shared Care Plan is available for free to anyone who wishes to use it. The full source code and complete documentation of the tool are available at http://www.peacehealth.org/scp. Anyone can download it. Hundreds of people all over the world have downloaded the code base and the documentation guide.

One question PeaceHealth staff is currently pondering is how its patient portal should interact with the Shared Care Plan and other PHRs. One idea is similar to the concept upon which Quicken (the financial management software) is based—that is, to try to standardize the systems so that a patient can interface his or her PHR with multiple organizational portals where patients may choose to receive services.

Gauthier concluded by saying that there is no shortage of great ideas from patients that then lead to new designs and built systems. The Shared Care Plan will keep evolving to incorporate those ideas.

OBSERVATIONS FROM THE EXAM ROOM: PATIENT-CENTERED HIT IMPLEMENTATION IN DIVERSE PRACTICE SETTINGS

Joshua Seidman, Ph.D., M.H.S.
President, Center for Information Therapy

Information therapy sits at the intersection of patient-centered care and health information technology (HIT). The Center for Information Therapy is an independent nonprofit organization whose mission is to advance the practice and the science of information therapy in order to improve people's health. The vision of the center is a future in which every health decision is informed.[7]

The center uses the logo "Ix" because Ix is a corollary to Rx, the standard symbol for a medical treatment or prescription. People talk about all the information that is available on the Web and, in general, it is positive that consumers have access to that information. But too much information

---

[7] The Center for Information Therapy website is www.ixcenter.org.

can create an information overdose. If people access inaccurate or incorrect information, that too can have negative side effects. Therefore, the issue can be seen as a matter of titrating the dosage of information. How does one figure out the appropriate dose, frequency, and duration of the information to provide? How can the right information be delivered to the right people at the right time so that they can better manage their health and make better health decisions?

Kerr White, an epidemiologist, developed the idea of the ecology of health care and medicine (1961). His idea was to examine a population of 1,000 people to determine how people experience health and health issues and how they use the health care system. This research was updated by Larry Green (a family physician) and colleagues (2001).

Green and his colleagues found that in a population of 1,000 people, on average about 800 would report symptoms of one sort or another. Of those reporting symptoms, 217 would visit a physician's office (including 113 who would visit a primary care physician), 65 would visit a complementary or alternative medicine provider, 21 would visit a hospital outpatient clinic, 14 would choose to receive home health care, 13 would visit an emergency department, and 8 would be hospitalized (with fewer than 1, on average, hospitalized in an academic medical center). There is a big difference between the number of people reporting symptoms and the number who actually seek care.

How does use of the Internet for seeking health information fit into this picture? Of those 1,000 people, it is known that considerably more than the number who seek care, but probably less than the 800 who report symptoms, will access the Internet for health information. There are different degrees of access to the Internet—some people have access at home, others at work, and still others have access through a family member. The Pew Internet and American Life Project found that 60 percent of people with household incomes below $40,000 per year had access to the Internet (Esterbrook et al., 2007).

More people now go online for health information every day than visit a doctor, which is what Susannah Fox of the Pew Internet and American Life Project referred to as the "Dr. Google" phenomenon. That raises the obvious question, What happens when physicians tell their patients not to go online? When surveyed on this question, consumers said that they either change where they are going for medical care or else just no longer tell their physicians about it (Fox and Fallows, 2003).

If one asks consumers where they would prefer to obtain information, they report that their first choice is from their personal physician. But when they do see their physician, the visit is often carried out in a very condensed timeframe with insufficient time to discuss everything they would like to talk about. Furthermore, about 50 to 80 percent of things a patient hears in the physician's office is completely forgotten by the time he or she gets home (Eiser, 1982) When the patient returns home, he or she will generally have numerous questions still unanswered. In response, the patient goes to the Internet. The patient may also go to other places as well in the search for information.

It is not difficult to find information on the Internet. The difficulty is finding information relative to a specific need. Even if people find what they need, they may not understand what they find. If they find and understand the information, the next challenge is to remember it. If they find, understand, and remember the information, they must then figure out how to contextualize it, that is, they must determine what the information means for their particular care and needs.

This is the task of information therapy; to figure out how to bring two worlds together in order to make sure that the information people need is there for them at the right time. Information therapy recognizes that there is a difference between data and information. If one looks at a PHR, for example, it may contain data that are hard to read and interpret. But going from data to information therapy requires making sense of those data and putting them into some context that leads to information, then to knowledge, and ultimately, to behavior.

Appropriate use of HIT can help individuals make informed health decisions. The Center for Information Therapy took part in a project that observed how clinicians and patients use HIT to advance patient education and to make better use of HIT tools.[8] Time was spent in a wide variety of settings—small practices with one or two physicians, for example, multi-specialty groups, and in integrated delivery systems. About half of the time was spent in federally qualified community health centers.

Health literacy issues cut across various populations. One important observation of the project was that some of the biggest health literacy challenges occur with people who have significantly impaired cognitive function, such as people with mental illness.

If one is to understand what actually happens with patients, one must spend time on site. For that reason, project staff spent a great deal of time observing the interactions of clinicians and patients. But before they observed these clinician/patient interactions, the project staff spoke with administrators of the facilities. One finding was that the way in which administrators viewed things was often contradicted by what

---

[8] Safety net providers observed included the Institute for Family Health (New York); East Boston Neighborhood Health Center; Cambridge Health Alliance (Massachusetts); La Clinica de La Raza (California); District of Columbia Primary Care Association; Lifelong Medical Care (California); Queens Health Network (New York); UNITE HERE! (New York); Urban Health Plan (New York); Baltimore Medical System; Redwood Community Health Coalition; and MiVia/La Luz Community Center (California).

actually was happening. In one community health center, for example, the chief information officer told the project staff, "Oh, we don't really need a PHR because our patients don't really want to access information electronically." But when the staff observed the primary care physician serving his patients over a 2-hour period, the physician received e-mails and text messages from patients on his cell phone. It turned out that the clinician's patients already were using electronic technology, but the message was not getting to the administrators of the center. Rather than making assumptions about what technologies patients do or do not use, one should use data and observations to determine what is actually occurring.

The project found that there was a great deal of variability in terms of the technology that patients were using. For example, in one inner-city community health center with a population that was about 95 percent Latino, the clinicians said, "All our patients use e-mail." In other communities patients were using smartcards. These smartcards contain patient information which can by read by smartcard readers at health care facilities in order to quickly obtain information about the patient. The smartcard readers cost about $15, so this approach is fairly inexpensive to implement. The problem is that facilities frequently do not plan in advance to buy smartcard readers when they buy their computers.

Similarly, many facilities are implementing electronic health records without thinking about the portal access. Furthermore, planning for PHRs is often done without thinking about the link between an individual's health information (e.g., a person's lab data, medical record, and medication information) and the context within which that information will be used. This is a serious concern, and it is important to think carefully about the best way to contextualize content. There is a great opportunity to do things correctly the first time, to make sure electronic records are patient-centered, as PeaceHealth and MiVIA have done.

There are many instances when PHRs are implemented but not much used. Providers don't promote their use or they may even object to their use—as in the case that Gauthier spoke of earlier where the physician threw the Shared Care Plan card in the trash. Patients need to be engaged, but clinicians must also be active participants in the process because patients do pay attention to what their clinicians say and give it a great deal of weight.

Observation shows that people are hungry for information but do not have very high expectations. As mentioned in earlier presentations, people need a reason to use technology. Once they have an experience of value to them, they are much more likely to use the technology. For example, technologies could create after-visit summaries in English, Spanish, or other languages. Given that patients forget 50 percent to 80 percent of what they hear in a physicians office (Eiser, 1982), such summaries could have a big effect on how the patients view technology.

A major challenge is the reimbursement system and the way that incentives are structured. Currently, particularly for community health centers, the in-person visit is the major source of income. But if technology use decreases the number of visits, it also decreases income. This issue must be addressed.

Crossing the Quality Chasm stated that health care in the past has been based on episodic encounters with the delivery system (IOM, 2001). It is important to create a system with a more continuous cycle of care and continuous healing relationships. Furthermore, as the report states, the system should encourage "all types of health care interactions that improve information transfer." On average, a patient's visit to a clinician lasts 16 minutes, during which the conversation between clinician and patient may cover six topics (Blumenthal et al., 1999). Information therapy and patient-centered HIT can help patients maximize the value of these visits by, for example, allowing them to obtain information in advance of the visit. By using HIT to obtain information in advance, the patient has a better sense of what might be expected, which sets the stage for more efficient use of time during the encounter. An after-visit summary would then reinforce what went on during the visit.

Seidman concluded by saying that use of PHRs increases ongoing communication for risk reduction, health promotion, care management, and, ultimately, decision support, particularly concerning high-end procedures. The Center for Information Therapy's annual meeting will explore HIT and patient-centered care as well as information therapy and health disparities, plus information therapy and health literacy.

DISCUSSION

George Isham, M.D., M.S.
HealthPartners
Moderator

An audience member said that what has been presented certainly has implications for building the medical home. The challenge will be to involve patients. Gauthier responded that in the PeaceHealth project participating clinics were often the first ones to introduce the concept of the Shared Care Plan and its personal health record to patients. They would display tent cards on their desks and stickers on their windows that said, "We support the Shared Care Plan." That advocacy for the personal health record helped convince patients.

Solomon said that MiVIA is actually the medical home for the people it serves because those members have so many providers. A member may go to a public health clinic, an emergency room, and two or three clinics in a just a few months. If the patient's health information is dispersed throughout all those sites, it can contribute to poor outcomes for the member. MiVIA, as a single storage site, can facilitate better coordination and outcomes. This does not mean that the various facilities do not have their own charts, but all the information relevant to the member is stored in the MiVIA personal health record.

The same participant asked what the repercussions are regarding reimbursement and revenue streams for using these electronic tools, especially for the providers who are providing clinical care.

Solomon replied that, for MiVIA, the members are mostly uninsured and use clinics that are reimbursed under special programs. It is critical, however, to start looking at how to promote reimbursement to providers so that they participate as partners with their patients in getting this information online. PHRs, especially with vulnerable populations, contribute to costs savings because results of tests are located in the record, which negates the need for running the same test or for scanning multiple times as the patient visits multiple providers.

One participant said that hearing about the Shared Care Plan is awe inspiring. How applicable is it to other parts of the country? The Shared Care Plan is in a rural area with a defined set of providers, and the patient research was conducted in that community. What can be learned from that work to think about how to apply this in other places?

Gauthier responded that the circumstances in Whatcom County did enable the project to move farther than, perhaps, other locales would. What was done in Whatcom County is available for download, but what is of foremost importance is that those constructing PHRs should conduct user research. One may or may not end up with the same kind of PHR that Whatcom County did. Certainly the example of MiVIA shows that things vary from city to city.

Another very important lesson is to give patients the respect they deserve for what they are trying to accomplish in the health care system. Many people have the attitude that getting clinicians together in a room to brainstorm about what patients need is sufficient, but that is simply not true. Just because a clinician works with patients on a day-to-day basis does not mean that the clinician understands what patients are experiencing at the pharmacy or when they go home.

Another useful thing would be to standardize the definition of a personal health record and the components that make up that record. Solomon said that the Markle Foundation, as part of its Connecting for Health work (http://www.connectingforhealth.org/workinggroups/personal healthwg.html), will be releasing some recommendations, principles, and policies regarding personal health information and the term "network PHRs." The technology is fast developing to the point where, given standards, one should be able to take a PHR from one system to another and share information.

In terms of usability in separate locations, MiVIA has been implemented not only on the West Coast but also in New York. Two networks that have migrant streams that go from New York to Florida are enrolling the members in New York and then having the clinics in Florida connect with those in New York.

But the most important things, Solomon continued, are first to educate, then to engage in outreach, and finally to proceed with implementation. One needs to educate the public and the provider communities about how PHR and technology can help. Next, outreach with communities and providers must be undertaken. Finally, one must implement the program.

One audience member said that, given the discussion, it seems correct to say that there is no standard PHR design or dominant design in the country. Is there a standard interface with electronic medical records?

Solomon responded that a standard interface is emerging. Just as CCHIT (Certification Commission for Healthcare Information Technology) offers certification for electronic medical records, HL7[9] will soon be releasing recommendations for interfaces around certain parts of the PHR. Standardization could happen, although it has not yet been accomplished. Information can be downloaded from the HL7 website at www.hl7.org.

Gauthier added that there are definitely opportunities for standardizing personal health records, but there will always be a need for segmentation. For example, a patient could take an activation quiz to find out where he or she is on the health literacy scale and then be prescribed a certain type of PHR based on how health-literate that patient is. As the patient progresses in health literacy, he or she could easily move information to a different PHR. That is where standards would be key.

Solomon was asked whether she thought that at some point any commercial application of EHR in the country would be able to feed MiVIA data. Absolutely, Solomon responded. MiVIA is already working with two electronic medical record companies and with other PHRs to accomplish this.

One questioner asked whether, within the MiVIA PHR design, there are any standards for the way information is displayed, for the level or

---

[9] "Health Level Seven is one of several American National Standards Institute (ANSI)-accredited Standards Developing Organizations (SDOs) operating in the healthcare arena. Health Level Seven's domain is clinical and administrative data" (Health Level Seven Inc., 2008).

density of text, or for readability levels of charts or information. This would seem to be important given the differing abilities of people to read and comprehend. Or is this an issue that people are just beginning to realize is important?

Solomon responded that this is an important issue. MiVIA has focused on technology, privacy, and security of applications. This third generation needs to start looking at health-literacy aspects.

One participant, noting that several of the speakers touched on training and helping people understand how to use the technology, asked, Are there any best practices or standards for how to do that effectively or well, or is it so early that one is just at the point of doing something and sharing information?

Gauthier responded that it has been her experience that people do not expect or want to have to go through a 2-hour training session to use a website. People expect to be able to sit down and use any website that is out there. With the newer technologies—for example, the so-called Ajax Rich Internet Applications—there is an opportunity to build robust contextual help. Patients may be listing their care team on the form with no problem, but then they get to the advanced directions and are at a loss for what to do. It is at this point that they are ready for a training module embedded in the application that could walk them through the process. Embedding more contextual training in the applications themselves is probably the best approach to take.

Seidman agreed, although he pointed out that there is a portion of the population that is not yet versed in computers and does not use them. The idea of using *promotores* or community health workers as educators is a good one which seems to work well. There are other resources that can be deployed as well, such as librarians and other ancillary health professionals. In many cases, however, it is the community health workers who have been found to be most effective and the best use of resources. In one case, for example, a janitor's union engaged unemployed janitors to help train union members in the use of computers. Union members' reception of the training was very positive.

Solomon remarked that, on average, it takes a physician anywhere from 4 to 12 hours to learn to use an electronic medical record. Outreach and training for the community using the *promotores* engages the members and is a good model. Such training is really health advocacy. During the session members learn about all kinds of things, including how to talk with the physician, how health care is important to the member, and the importance of the member being a partner in the health care experience.

One audience member said that it is important that those designing PHRs want to listen—to hear from the patients about their needs. Starting with people's needs and working with them is crucial. But how does one make that grow? Are there ways to use these approaches in adult education or in K-12 education to involve the next generation in skill building around use of these technological tools and to learn about the kinds of chronic conditions one might have, the immunizations one needs, and the medicines one takes? Another alternative might be to work with large employers and labor to engage populations in understanding information about their health and how to act on such information.

Solomon responded that one of the successful things MiVIA did was to create a curriculum called the Student Health Ambassadorship Program. MiVIA representatives visited the local high school and, through the high school principal, recruited three ESL (English as a Second Language) students. For 3 months, these students met once a week for about 2 hours to learn about information technology, health advocacy and bilingual assistance. They worked with the outreach workers as well. One of these students was a shy young lady about 16 years old who would not look at anyone directly. That young lady is now a sophomore in college, focusing on health care. She has created her own curriculum and is working with PTAs (parent-teacher associations), the councils, and with teachers at various schools. Patient navigators or student health ambassadors are an important tool.

Seidman said that working with *promotores* and community health workers to train people in the use of the Internet also creates other social and employment opportunities. He described his experience as a volunteer and president of the board of directors of a transitional house for homeless women in recovery from substance abuse in the mid- and late 1990s. At that time computers and the Internet were just beginning to emerge as being of major importance to individuals, and his group realized that women wanted to develop their skills with the computer. The board bought a computer for the house, and it became an important benefit for the women living there as they created their independent lives. Creating these kinds of opportunities is something that should be kept in mind.

Isham concluded the discussion by stating that the presentations and conversations had been excellent in terms of helping the audience realize that there is an interesting interface between health literacy and technology that needs to be explored. It is not clear, however, that most of those engaged in developing these technological tools are currently aware of or exploring that interface.

5

Emerging Tools and Strategies

A GUIDE FOR DEVELOPING AND PURCHASING SUCCESSFUL HEALTH INFORMATION TECHNOLOGY

Cindy Brach, M.P.P.
Senior Health Policy Researcher,
Agency for Healthcare Research and Quality

The Agency for Healthcare Research and Quality (AHRQ) is a leader in the field of health information technology (HIT). It has an extensive HIT portfolio and operates the National Resource Center (NRC)[1] for HIT. Previous speakers have noted that there is not a great deal of awareness about health literacy issues in the IT world and that we need to raise that level of awareness. As an evidence-based agency, AHRQ wants to put forward what is known in the field about better ways of developing HIT that will lead to more effective ways to communicate effectively with all audiences.

The NRC was asked to develop a health literacy guide for HIT developers and purchasers. The project was managed jointly by Prashila

---

[1] NORC (the National Opinion Research Center), "in cooperation with several partners, has led the development of a national resource center (NRC) for AHRQ's Health Information Technology (health IT) initiative. The AHRQ NRC supports over 100 AHRQ HIT grantees, five State and Regional Demonstration (SRD) projects working toward health information exchange, as well as 33 states and one territory working on a Health Information Security and Privacy Collaboration" (National Opinion Research Center, 2008).

Dullabh and June Eichner. The goal of the guide is to assist developers, the people who are creating new software programs, to become more aware of and more knowledgeable about health literacy issues. For purchasers, the guide includes a checklist of things they should look for when evaluating whether to buy a particular HIT product.

The project first reviewed the literature, both the IT and HIT literature, to find out what was known about ways to develop health information technology so that it would be accessible to limited-literacy audiences. Project staff also looked at various products and websites such as MiVIA. Finally, project staff held discussions with individuals who develop and purchase HIT as well as with researchers involved in the evaluation of HIT for limited literacy populations.

Not surprisingly, the literature on developing accessible health information technology for limited-literacy audiences is scanty; very little has been published about the best way to proceed. As discussed in this workshop, there may not be a single "best" way; instead systems should be adapted to a particular community or population.

AHRQ views health information technology as including personal health records, electronic health records, and health information exchange. The guide covers a number of different types of technology that can be used to convey health information to various audiences, including Internet websites, touch screen kiosks, personal wireless devices (e.g., cell phones, BlackBerrys, and personal digital assistants or PDAs), and home monitoring devices.

The guide promotes the use of universal basic design principles. First, use a simple structure with clean looks that highlight important elements. Second, build well, taking advantage of the technology inherent in the application in order to give consumers choices. Finally, for Internet sites, it is important to use HTML rather than other formats because HTML is more accessible to consumers.

An example of a simple design is shown in Figure 5-1. This design, which is still in testing, is a version of an update to prevention information in healthfinder.gov, which has been attempting to find which approaches are more responsive to and work best for consumers. As can be seen, the design contains only five headings of two or three words each: (1) Eat Healthy, (2) Get Active, (3) Get Screened, (4) Quit Smoking, and (5) Watch Your Weight. Each of the subsequent Web pages takes a similarly clean approach, presenting quite a bit of information but in a clear, simple, and understandable way.

Much of the guide[2] adheres to current guidelines for print materials.

---

[2] The guide is called *Accessible Health Information Technology (IT) for Populations with Limited Literacy: A Guide for Developers and Purchasers of Health IT*. It is available on AHRQ's National

EMERGING TOOLS AND STRATEGIES   75

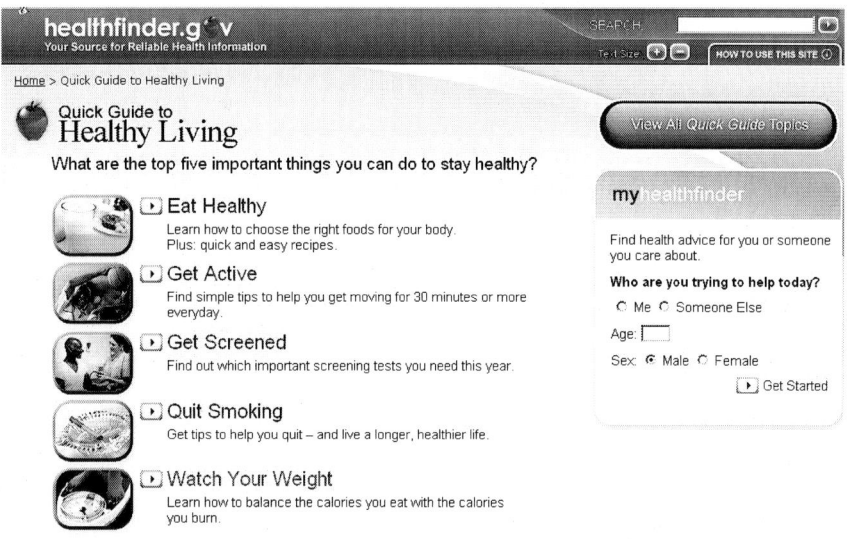

FIGURE 5-1 Simple design.
SOURCE: Brach, 2008.

For example, the content should assume that the browser has little or no background knowledge, information should be relevant to users, it should deliver a limited number of messages, and it should use numbers and percentages that are appropriate. Furthermore, one should use graphics only if they clarify text. There should be white space, lines should be short, and text should be broken up and chunked. Text should be in a large and familiar dark font on a light background, and there should be a consistent use of font sizes and styles with both upper and lower case letters, and justification to the left-hand margin only.

It is also important to develop content that is culturally competent. Guidelines for cultural competence require content that is culturally appropriate and sensitive to users, and that members of groups be portrayed accurately in pictures and other graphic illustrations. The guidelines also require that translation from English be accurate and that idioms and expressions be appropriate.

Iterative testing is critical. The recommended process is to draft a prototype, conduct a team review and a review by health-literacy experts,

---

Resource Center for Health Information Technology at http://healthit.ahrq.gov/portal/server.pt/gateway/PTARGS_0_3882_803031_0_0_18/LiteracyGuide.pdf.

and then revise the prototype based on the results of that review. After that, the revised design should be tested with a target audience that is culturally diverse and that includes limited-literacy members. During the test the audience should be observed using the technology, they should be asked about their experiences, and their comprehension should be assessed. Based on this test, the technology should be revised again and, if the technology will be in multiple languages, it should be tested in all those languages as well.

Some considerations are specific to HIT. For example, design needs to be usable with both old and new hardware and software. Some users may have black and white monitors, some may have slow Internet connections that would take a very long time to load fancy images, and some may not have the plug-ins needed to access complicated graphics. The home page of the website must be simple, and information should be prioritized with a minimal amount of text per screen. Furthermore, it is important that navigation is simple and consistent, with minimal need for scrolling. Limited-literacy individuals often have great difficulty with the concept that they have to scroll down to obtain more information. AHRQ frequently uses the three-click rule, that is, one must get users to the information in three clicks or face the possibility of losing them.

Searching must be simplified, as it is one of the more difficult operations for individuals with limited literacy. They frequently misspell words, and they may find it difficult to understand the search engines. The site should have clearly defined hyperlinks and a printer-friendly option. Audio transcription is an option to consider, especially for people who have difficulty reading or seeing, as well as for those who have a hard time finding information, particularly such things as instructions for using home health equipment. It is also a good idea to give users information about how to call for assistance.

Certain lessons have been learned about the use of computer kiosks. For example, it is important to have a practice session to familiarize users with the eLearning method. There should be one idea or question per screen and information should be limited to what is needed to manage the health problem. There should also be an option that allows the user to repeat a message and there should be some kind of teach-back built in so that learning can be reinforced. Again, audio transcription should be considered.

The guide also discusses personal wireless devices. When developing programs for these devices for use by adults with limited literacy, reliance on text should be minimized, and text messaging should be simplified.

There are a number of ways to make home monitoring devices such as glucometers and blood pressure cuffs easier to use including limiting the number of steps needed to use the device, using large keys with clear icons, including a self-calculating feature, and adding voice instructions and results. Clear presentation of results is important. For example, a person with limited literacy will find it easier to understand a message that says "Your blood sugar is too high" than one that provides a number that must be interpreted. Instructions should be clear and easy to follow, using simple print and video tutorials with illustrations for each step of use. One should avoid very small fonts and technical medical language, for instance. Critical components or warnings should be emphasized.

Brach concluded by saying that, in thinking about the future it is important to start incorporating literacy and health literacy considerations into the development of personal health records and ePrescribing.

DISCUSSION

George Isham, M.D., M.S.
HealthPartners
Moderator

One audience member said that many of her patients who use the Internet have difficulty so they look for a telephone number to call to obtain assistance. Yet, she said, it is usually not possible to find a telephone number. The audience member urged AHRQ to be careful about posting guidelines on telephone use if there is not someone available to receive calls. Brach agreed that it was important to have someone available to answer calls.

Another participant asked if Brach could elaborate on what she meant when she talked about making information culturally relevant. Brach responded that some of the things one might look for are whether the graphics are relevant to the population. Unfortunately, there is not a science base that one can point to and say, if one follows this checklist, one will be culturally competent. It is a very complex issue.

Another audience member pointed out that there does not seem to be a consensus about what the three to five actionable items are that could lead to quality improvement in various areas. What is it that everyone needs to know how to do in order to improve diabetes outcomes, for example, or asthma outcomes? It is a great deal easier to build platforms for communicating if one agrees on the actionable points. Any leadership or guidance that AHRQ can provide on how to do a better job of coming up with some common consensus about what one needs to know about health literacy would be very helpful.

Brach responded that AHRQ and those in the Department of Health and Human Services (HHS) working on healthfinder.gov have been in the process of building consensus on the top prevention and health promotion messages. They started with an exhaustive search of all HHS documents and have winnowed the material down to five messages. So there is recognition that this is an important avenue to pursue.

One audience member asked if AHRQ is tracking who is asking for and using the health literacy guide and if there are plans to determine whether or not the guide makes a difference. Brach responded that AHRQ tracks the number of hits and downloads of the document, but it cannot collect information about who is using the guide and what their experience is. It might be possible to conduct a study to examine those issues.

HEALTH LITERACY, HEALTH INFORMATION TECHNOLOGY, AND HEALTHY PEOPLE 2020

Linda Harris, Ph.D.
Lead, Health Communication and eHealth Team
Office of Disease Prevention and Health Promotion

Charles P. Friedman, Ph.D.
Deputy National Coordinator for
Health Information Technology
Department of Health and Human Services

Healthy People is a comprehensive set of national 10-year objectives that provide a framework for public health priorities and actions, Harris explained. As many know, Healthy People 2010 has a communication focus and, within that focus, one of the objectives is to improve and address limited health literacy. Other topics in the 2010 communication focus area are meaningful access to the Internet, health website quality, research-based health communication with an evaluation component, and supporting patient-provider communication.

Planning for the Healthy People 2020 is now under way, with the mission, the vision, and the objectives yet to be defined. Work began in 2005 with meetings of experts to provide suggestions for how it should be organized. In 2007 this group presented its ideas. The year 2008 has been and will continue to be focused on building a framework for Healthy People 2020. During 2009, measurable objectives will be developed and, in 2010, Healthy People 2020 will be launched.

The group of experts involved in the planning of Healthy People 2020 presented a different approach from the alphabetical categorization of objectives in Healthy People 2010, proposing two major focus areas. The current idea is that the primary focus would be on risk factors and determinants of health, that is, on the primary factors related to health and disparities. The secondary focus would be on diseases and disorders.

The intent is that Healthy People 2020 create a systems view of health, to organize it around different contexts and different important factors. There are three high priorities in public health. First is prevention, second is preparedness, and third is HIT.

In late 2007, the Office of Disease Prevention and Health Promotion, the Office of the National Coordinator for Health Information Technology, and the Centers for Disease Control and Prevention (CDC) formed a federal interagency subgroup on health communication and information technology. The purpose of the group is to create a vision and project a future in which health communication and information technologies significantly advance the goals of Healthy People 2020. Public forums, a blog and a wiki will provide an opportunity for input from the public about how health literacy is important and the role that health literacy should play in the development of the framework for Healthy People 2020.

Friedman said that it is fascinating, exciting, and an enormous challenge to combine health literacy, health information technology, and health communications as a major foundational element of the Healthy People 2020 activity. The Office of the National Coordinator (ONC) for Health Information Technology, in collaboration with a large number of people, has been working to conceptualize a vision of what information technology might look like in the future and to develop a national 5-year HIT strategic plan (2008 to 2012). Efforts in this area began in 2007 and the plan is in the final stages of federal clearance.[3] The plan has two broad goals. The first goal centers on person-focused health care. In addition to discussing the hardware and software aspects of IT, much of what is discussed in the plan will address the person–focused aspects of health care. Furthermore, the plan envisions IT as a means to achieve a healthier population.

A second goal concerns the improvement of population health. The plan defines population health as having four components: public health, preparedness, biomedical research, and health care quality improvement. The plan is national in scope and is federally focused, setting forth a set of strategies that can be undertaken across a broad range of federal agencies.

Each of the two goals in the plan has four objectives with measurable outcomes. For the eight objectives there are a total of 43 strategies listed, each with a milestone. Some of the milestones are near-term (i.e., 2009 or 2010), while others are longer-term (i.e., 2011 or 2012). Perhaps the most important feature of the plan is that it will include a compendium of federal activities already under way that are related to the various objectives of the plan and that are taking place in the agencies and departments involved in putting the plan together.

---

[3] The *ONC-Coordinated Federal HIT Strategic Plan: 2008-2012* was released June 3, 2008.

Harris said that the Federal Interagency Advisory Group will be the decision maker for Healthy People 2020. Current members of the group include only agencies from HHS, but the membership will soon expand to other agencies. As mentioned earlier, there is a Health Communication and Health Information Technology subgroup. The group's task is to determine how health communication, health literacy, and HIT can provide an infrastructure for the achievement of Healthy People 2020. The strategic thinking presented in the ONC strategic plan will be woven throughout the work of this subgroup. Questions to be addressed include, What should be measured in health literacy and how should that be measured?

Harris concluded by saying that an effort to envision the future of an integrated system of health literacy, health communication, and HIT has begun. The subgroup will be advising the Secretary of HHS. Input is needed from those who are expert in the area of health literacy as well as from the public in general.

DISCUSSION

George Isham, M.D., M.S.
HealthPartners
Moderator

One audience member from a private health system said that his system has had a series of 5-year goals and each time it prepared for the next set, the system attempted to evaluate what had been learned from the previous set of goals. What information from Healthy People 2010, he asked, is being used as input to Healthy People 2020 in terms of the communication objectives and, more specifically, health literacy? Harris responded that it is not clear that Healthy People 2020 should measure the same things that Healthy People 2010 measured. At present the health literacy of the population is being measured. But if one thinks in terms of infrastructure, one could measure other things, such as how many physicians are trained in health literacy. One might set an objective to have all providers obtain continuing medical education credit for health communication or health literacy training. This is the kind of objective that could be incorporated into Healthy People if one thinks of it as representing an integrated infrastructure with skills, tools, and best practices.

Friedman asked for input from members of the audience about whether they believed that Healthy People 2020 should include objectives directly related to HIT, health literacy, or health communication or whether those three components should be viewed in a more integrated fashion as a means to an end. One audience member replied that objectives should relate directly to health literacy. The bottom line is that what is measured is what gets done. Low health literacy has been a barrier to many improvements in health. To create the correct incentives, one must measure the correct things, so only if there is an explicit focus on health literacy will people address its issues.

One audience member said that it appeared to him that a set of goals for the nation must be anchored in improving the health of the population. Many things are enabling factors to improving the health of the citizens of the United States. Ultimately, however, the goals must lead to improving the health of the population. How one thinks about that is informed by one's experience over time. The government has been engaged in this effort for 40 years now, and this will be the third decade of the iteration of these goals. What specifically is being learned from what has happened in the past?

An audience member noted that there is an Institute of Medicine report on health literacy that made a number of recommendations (IOM, 2004). It would probably be helpful to review those recommendations and determine the kind of progress achieved for the recommendations related to the communications and health objectives of Healthy People 2020.

Another participant asked if the primary goal or vision of Healthy People 2020 is as global as improving the health of the nation or is more specifically focused on reducing disparities. Health information technology is very broad. Health communication, being about health information and its transfer, is a bit more specific. And health literacy is about what people understand and what they can do with the information they have been given. Will Healthy People 2020 attempt to weave these three things together to improve health or to reduce disparities?

Harris responded that Healthy People 2020 is about both improving the health of the population and reducing disparities. Health communication and HIT will have to be able to address both. Friedman said that they are attempting to mix three different cultures—HIT, health communication, and health literacy—that have similar problems and issues but that have addressed them in different ways. The challenge is to integrate the fundamentally different approaches that these three groups take to address problems. If successful, there will be a synergy that creates a whole far greater than the sum of its parts.

The Health Communication and Health Information Technology subgroup is inviting people who represent these three domains to work together. The hope is that through a combination of interaction and analysis a synergistic product will emerge. Perhaps in 2008 it is possible for these domains to function separately, but by 2020 it is likely that the groups will have had to merge.

When addressing the issue of who is missing from the discussion of health literacy, one audience member suggested that the behavior side of the equation is less prominent than it could be. A major goal is to motivate behavior change that will lead to improved health. However the people who are experts in behavior modification and behavior change don't seem to have played a major role.

Harris responded that, at is core, Healthy People is a stakeholder-driven effort. The groups organizing it are made up of federal government people. But there is an important forum for the public and for professionals to put forth their ideas about what Healthy People 2020 should look like. Friedman stated that it is often said in health informatics that the field is 80 percent about psychology and sociology and 20 percent about technology. It may be that individuals are attracted to the field because it is more about people and changing the way they work in a positive way than it is about software and hardware.

One audience member said that one of the specific objectives in the health communication goal of Healthy People 2010 was to increase individuals' health literacy. The National Assessment of Adult Literacy (NAAL) instrument was developed as a way of measuring this objective. Because there was measurement at only one point, however, it is not possible to determine whether individual health literacy has improved. Furthermore, the measure is about reading comprehension in a health context, which is not the same as health literacy. Dave Baker[4] says that health literacy is the interaction or the combination of what the individual brings to the situation and the demands placed on the individual, both the print and verbal demands. Much of the discussion and effort surrounding health literacy has focused on trying to reduce the demands.

Some of the other measures in Healthy People 2010 concern people's use of the Internet for health information. There is a graphic of the NAAL results that displays the amount of information that people get from the Internet by health literacy level. People with below basic levels of health literacy had very low rates of using the Internet and people in the proficient category had very high rates. This might be a good measure to use. IT could be measured again in 5 years to determine if there is an increase in people with limited literacy using the Internet for health information.

Another audience member asked whether we are accommodating or skill building. Accommodating is a legitimate strategy, but it needs to be recognized as such. One must also recognize that the determinants of health are very broad.

One participant asked how much of the IT conversation addresses

---

[4] David W. Baker wrote The meaning and the measure of health literacy. 2006. *Journal of General Internal Medicine: Official Journal of the Society for Research and Education in Primary Care Internal Medicine* 21(8):878-883.

population-level tools today versus a potential tomorrow. In Minnesota, for example, probably about 80 percent of the providers have HIT tools, but that is very different from the country overall.

It is also interesting, the participant continued, that HIT is not yet associated with performance. That is, having HIT is not yet a factor in terms of improving performance because many systems are old-school technologies. Perhaps there should be short-term and long-term objectives that address the progress in improving health, with old-school technologies being used while the infrastructure for IT is being built in order to enable something more in the future. It frequently is the case that things take longer to occur than one envisions, so it may be that the benefits of IT will take much longer to achieve. If one places a great deal of emphasis on IT in Healthy People 2020, one may not actually make a lot of progress in improving the nation's health in the interim.

Another participant stated that IT can, if developed with more than just a focus on the individual, facilitate examination of population-level health. How do the risk factors as determinants of health relate to the infrastructure IT issues? Friedman agreed that it is important to focus on population HIT tools.

Harris replied that that is part of the framework development that the groups are working on. How might they relate to one another? Also, for the first time, there is public advisory group that is providing input to the Secretary. Jonathan Fielding is chair of that 13-member group which will also be discussing these issues and questions. There is a dialogue between the federal interagency group and the public advisory group. A public comment page has been added to the Healthy People website and everyone is urged to ask questions and make comments.

One audience member said that 10 years from now it will likely be possible to measure genetic risk factors for various populations in order to judge which interventions will work best for which populations. Will Healthy People 2020 address genetics? Friedman responded that this is one of the areas that, as an audience member observed earlier, will probably take longer to achieve than is currently anticipated.

Another audience member said that many people still do not understand health literacy or its importance for health. Healthy People is an important effort that could help bring much needed attention to the issues of health literacy and its affect on health. One may say that health literacy is a tool that flows across objectives, but if there are not explicit objectives related to health literacy, important stakeholders will be missing from the discussion and action. Health literacy is a determinant of health, one which will be of even more importance by 2020. The participant concluded by saying that including specific health literacy objectives in Healthy People would place a national focus on this important area.

6

Concluding Discussion

George Isham, M.D., M.S.
HealthPartners
Moderator

The audience was asked to reflect on the entire workshop and to ask questions of any of the speakers who presented during the day.

One participant remarked that the lack of standardization of personal health records (PHRs) and electronic health records (EHRs) is fascinating. It is encouraging that there are efforts to develop standards for the interface of these two and there appears to be a great deal of opportunity for developing display approaches and tools that address some health literacy concerns. Yet there is much that is unknown about how a range of people with differing skill levels and different education levels can understand and effectively use these tools. A digital divide remains, with the people on the wrong side of the divide tending to be the people with poorer health status and poorer health outcomes. Gauthier's position that patient-centered care equals user-centered design is a great summary of what needs to be done, the participant concluded.

One participant commented that Susannah Fox suggests that, rather than thinking of Internet use in terms of a digital divide where everyone can be classified as being in one camp or another—like an on/off switch—it makes more sense to think of the situation in terms of a thermometer where everyone is on a continuum of use and everyone's use is increasing.

Another audience member said that she believes there is a need for standardization in the exchange of information among PHRs and between PHRs and the EHRs. However there is a danger in rushing too quickly to standardize before there is enough information about what is important. Another issue in standardization is that people's expectations and desires about how things look change over time. If there is not room for modification, people may not pay attention to a site or to the available information there.

Another participant noted that many of the presenters talked about the importance of obtaining user feedback and observing users, which is very important in the development of these health information technology (IT) systems.

Kukafka commented that while there may be a need for standards in terms of exchange between systems, there has been little discussion about tailoring or personalizing content, which is what the data and research indicate people find most salient. It appears that people today want something targeted specifically for them at the time they need it. If one can assess a person's literacy level, one can provide that person with exactly what he or she needs. One is spared the issues associated with population-based approaches to communication, issues such as whether one should present all information at a 6th-grade level. What happens when the information is at a 6th-grade level but the person accessing it is at the 12th-grade level? Does that put them off? In terms of improving health, providing individuals with tailored messages may well be a successful approach.

Tailoring and personalizing content are critical, Seidman agreed, not only because of issues such as health literacy, but also because content needs to be provided at the action level. For example, in attempting to get someone to quit smoking, providing information to that person if he or she is in the pre-contemplation stage will not be as effective.

Another issue, one participant said, is whether measurements should focus on process or outcome. That is, should one measure what needs to be learned concerning an individual's interaction with information technology, or should one measure whether the interaction between an individual and the technology resulted in that person doing what he or she should—for example, taking the medication appropriately? What does it take to get the proper reaction or behavior?

It was pointed out that many people using the Internet or other IT tools are not looking for information in order to take action. Instead they are trying to understand something they have just been told.

One participant said that in the broader eHealth world it does not appear that the people designing health information technology (HIT) systems have an understanding of the issues of health literacy or their importance. Yet there have been several presentations about development of systems that did focus on the health literacy needs of their users. Is there any guidance that the presenters can give about how to bring these issues to the broader eHealth world?

Marchibroda responded that, currently, health literacy is separate from the development of HIT systems. The focus is on putting electronic health records into physicians' offices and helping emergency rooms to obtain data. The focus is very provider-centric in other words, and there are many barriers to that adoption. Consumer-facing applications are happening in some areas—Whatcom County, for example—and personal record organizations are working directly with employers or health plans. To bring health literacy more broadly into the development of HIT requires addressing some of the barriers to implementation, particularly making the business case.

There are also other things that could be done, Marchibroda continued. The first is raising awareness of how important health literacy is in the development of these systems. The second is raising expectations of what is expected from providers in terms of health literacy. In terms of measurement, one might start with some process measures but what ultimately drives change is what is rewarded in health care. It is important to show that obtaining higher-quality health outcomes requires more effective consumer–clinician engagement and understanding.

The questioner responded that focusing on improving physician understanding of health literacy may result in the kind of situation that now exists with IT systems for prescription medications. That is, the systems are designed for ease of communication between the pharmacist and the physician, but that does not necessarily have anything to do with increasing patient understanding about taking medication.

Seidman said that there has been a great deal of conversation about health behavior change and how to get individuals to make different choices or to learn certain skills. But it is important to remember that people are embedded within communities and individual practitioners are embedded in organizations. Perhaps some of the largest gains could be made by looking at that bigger picture.

Systems are critical, he continued. Many approaches assume that everyone has the same advantages. However, those who are poor, unwell, or uneducated have many things working against them. For example, the action taken in the Arizona Medicaid program to give people e-mail addresses was a system action. Going to where people are rather then expecting individuals to take responsibility is a shift in organizational thinking. Such a shift would include creating health-promoting types of systems that help develop literacy cultures. The wiki has been discussed before. The power of the wiki is that there are a number of people working together, beyond the individual. One is actually tapping into the system in which those people are embedded.

One participant said that in order to make sure decent electronic health records are widespread one should work with the patients, the consumers, and the families. Health providers will demand integrated systems when patients arrive at their offices saying things like, "Here is my electronic health record. Why can't you download your standard information to me? Where are my MRIs? You should be able to e-mail those to me or put them on my thumb drive." The Commission on Systemic Interoperability took the position that more people need to demand interoperability. If that were done, health providers would be motivated to demand integrated systems.

Isham concluded the session by saying that many important questions remain about the integration of health literacy with developing HIT systems. For example, do the current methods used for assessing health literacy apply to the human–IT interface? There were many anecdotes throughout the day about how people interact with their machines and their PDAs and about how games are important. Are the NAALs and the other tools for assessing health literacy valid for assessing how effectively people understand and use information to improve health when that information is mediated through technology?

Another question for future exploration relates to the source of the $86.6 billion in savings spoken of earlier that it is estimated will be realized from the implementation of health care IT systems. While some might find it difficult to understand how such savings will accrue, it is likely that the interface between people and IT machines is a critical component in harvesting that savings. Perhaps if we understood that interface better, many would think that health literacy contributes more to savings than is currently realized and, therefore, would conclude that it is a much more important objective for Healthy People 2020 and other efforts.

References

2020 Systems. *2020 systems "Online marketing. Made easy,"* http://www.2020systems.com/internet-ad-glossary-r-z.html (accessed August 14, 2008).

AgrAbility Project. 2005. Health literacy: A critical but hidden health issue. *AgrAbility Quarterly* 6(1):2–4.

Ahern, D., J. Kreslake, and J. Phalen. 2006. What is eHealth (6): Perspectives on the evolution of eHealth research. *Journal of Medical Internet Research* 8(1):e4.

American Academy of Orthopedic Surgeons. 2007. *Discrepancy in healthcare utilization: Is more better in orthopedic surgery?* http://www.aaos.org/news/bulletin/jun07/reimbursement2.asp (accessed December 4, 2007).

American Library Association Presidential Committee on Information Literacy. 1989. *Final report.* Washington, DC: American Library Association.

Baldry, M., C. Cheal, B. Fisher, M. Gillett, and V. Huet. 1986. Giving patients their own records in general practice: Experience of patients and staff. *British Medical Journal (Clinical Research Edition)* 292(6520):596–598.

Bates, D., L. Leape, D. Cullen, N. Laird, L. Petersen, J. Teich, E. Burdick, M. Hickey, S. Kleefield, B. Shea, M. V. Vliet, and D. Seger. 1998. Effect of computerized physician order entry and a team intervention on prevention of serious medication errors. *JAMA* 280:1311–1316.

Berland, G., M. Elliott, and L. Morales. 2001. Health information on the internet: Accessibility, quality, and readability in English and Spanish. *JAMA* 285:2616–2621.

Blumenthal, D., N. Causino, Y. Chang, L. Culpepper, W. Marder, D. Saglam, R. Stafford, and B. Starfield. 1999. The duration of ambulatory visits to physicians. *Journal of Family Practice* 48(4):264–271.

Brach, C. 2008. *A guide for developing and purchasing successful health information technology.* Powerpoint presentation at the Institute of Medicine workshop on health literacy, eHealth, and communication: Putting the consumer first. Washington, DC, March 17.

CDC (Centers for Disease Control and Prevention). 2008. *Prevention research centers.* http://www.cdc.gov/prc/ (accessed August 14, 2008).

Colorado Department of Public Health and Environment. 2008. *Glossary of genetics terms.* http://www.cdphe.state.co.us/ps/genetics/glossary.html#M (accessed August 14, 2008).

Commonwealth Fund. 2006. *Why not the best?: Results from a national scorecard on US health system performance.* http://www.commonwealthfund.org/publications/publications_show.htm?doc_ id=401577 (accessed June 18, 2008).

Department of Veterans Affairs. 2008a. *Bar code medication administration (BCMA).* http://www.innovations.va.gov/innovations/page.cfm?pg=13 (accessed August 14, 2008).

Department of Veterans Affairs. 2008b. *Vista imaging.* http://www1.va.gov/imaging/ (accessed August 14, 2008).

Deutsche Telekom. 2008. *Group report, January 1 to March 31, 2006.* http://www.interimreport.telekom.de/site0106/en/co/glossar/index.php (accessed August 14, 2008).

Dewey, J. 1926. *Democracy and education: An introduction to the philosophy of education.* New York: Macmillan.

eHealth Initiative and Foundation for eHealth Initiative. 2008a. *eHealth initiative—about.* http://www.ehealthinitiative.org/about/ (accessed August 14, 2008).

eHealth Initiative and Foundation for eHealth Initiative. 2008b. *Fourth annual survey of information exchange at the state, regional, and community levels.* http://www.ehealthinitiative.org/2007HIESurvey/stateOfTheField.mspx#1 (accessed June 20, 2008).

eHealth Initiative and Foundation for eHealth Initiative. 2008c. *Results of 2008 Survey on Health Information Exchange: State of the Field.* http://www.ehealthinitiative.org/HIESurvey/2008State OfTheField.mspx. (accessed January 22, 2009).

Eiser, J. R. 1982. *Social psychology and behavioral medicine.* London: Wiley.

Eng, T., A. Maxfield, K. Patrick, M. Deering, S. Ratzan, and D. Gustafson. 1998. Access to health information and support: A public highway or a private road? *JAMA* 280:1371–1375.

Esterbrook, L., E. Witt, and L. Rainie. 2007. *Information searches that solve problems.* http://www.pewinternet.org/pdfs/Pew_UI_LibrariesReport.pdf (accessed July 17, 2008).

Fox, S. 2006. *Online health search 2006.* Washington, DC: Pew Internet and American Life Project.

Fox, S. 2007. *E-patients with a disability or chronic disease.* Washington, DC: Pew Internet and American Life Project.

Fox, S., and D. Fallows. 2003. *Internet health resources.* Washington, DC: Pew Internet and American Life Project.

Gauthier, D. 2008. *A user centered personal health record: The design and development of the shared care plan.* Powerpoint presentation at the Institute of Medicine workshop on health literacy, eHealth, and communication: Putting the consumer first. Washington, DC, March 17.

Governors State University. 2008. *eLearning.* http://www.govst.edu/elearning/default.aspx?id=12984 (accessed August 14, 2008).

Green, L., G. Fryer, B. Yawn, D. Lanier, and S. Dovey. 2001. Ecology of medical care revisited. *New England Journal of Medicine* 344:2021–2025.

Gross, L. 2006. Scientific illiteracy and the partisan takeover of biology. *PLoS Biology* 4(5): e167.

Health Level Seven Inc. 2008. *Health level 7.* http://www.hl7.org/ (accessed August 14, 2008).

Healthcare Information and Management Systems Society. 2005. *Personal health record.* http://www.himss.org/asp/topics_phr.asp (accessed August 14, 2008).

Healthwise. 2008. *Healthwise among the first to receive NCQA health information product certification.* http://hwinfo.healthwise.org/docs/DOCUMENT/9166.pdf (accessed August 14, 2008).

HHS (Department of Health and Human Services). 2006. *Four cornerstones of value driven health care.* http://www.hhs.gov/valuedriven/fourcornerstones/index.htm (accessed June 20, 2008).

Himmelstein, D., E. Warren, D. Thorne, and S. Woolhandler. 2005. Illness and injury as contributors to bankruptcy. *Health Affairs* 24:w63–w73.

Horrigan, J. 2006. *The internet as a resource for news and information about science.* Washington, DC: Pew Internet and American Life Project.

IOM (Institute of Medicine). 2000. *To err is human: Building a safer health system.* Washington, DC: National Academy Press.

IOM. 2001. *Crossing the quality chasm: A new health system for the 21st century.* Washington, DC: National Academy Press.

IOM. 2002. *Unequal treatment: Confronting racial and ethnic disparities in health care.* Washington, DC: The National Academies Press.

IOM. 2003. *Key capabilities of an electronic health record system.* Washington, DC: The National Academies Press.

IOM. 2004. *Health literacy: A prescription to end confusion.* Washington, DC: The National Academies Press.

IOM. 2007. *Preventing medication errors.* Washington, DC: The National Academies Press.

Johnston, D., E. Pan, B. Middleton, J. Walker, and D. Bates. 2003. *The value of computerized provider order entry in ambulatory settings.* Boston, MA: Center for Information Technology Leadership.

Jupitermedia Corporation. 2008. *ISP glossary.* http://isp.webopedia.com/TERM/W/wireframe.html (accessed August 14, 2008).

Kaiser Family Foundation and Health Research and Educational Trust. 2006. *Employer health benefits 2006 annual survey.* http://www.kff.org/insurance/7527/ (accessed June 18, 2008).

Kukafka, R. 2008. *Internet approaches for eHealth in low literacy and limited English proficiency populations.* Powerpoint presentation at the Institute of Medicine workshop on health literacy, eHealth, and communication: Putting the consumer first. Washington, DC, March 17.

Laugksch, R. 2000. Scientific literacy: A conceptual overview. *Science Education* 84:71–94.

Logan, R. 2000. *The sixth language: Learning a living in the internet age.* Toronto, ON: Stoddart Publications

Marchibroda, J. M. 2008. *Overview of eHealth.* Powerpoint presentation at the Institute of Medicine workshop on health literacy, eHealth, and communication: Putting the consumer first. Washington, DC, March 17.

MariosAlexandrou.com. 2008. *Definition of web portal.* http://www.mariosalexandrou.com/definition/web-portal.asp (accessed August 14, 2008).

Markle Foundation. 2005. *Attitudes of Americans regarding personal health records and nationwide electronic health information exchange: Key findings from two surveys of Americans.* Alexandria, VA: Public Opinion Strategies.

McGlynn, E. A., S. M. Asch, J. Adams, J. Keesey, J. Hicks, A. DeCristofaro, and E. A. Kerr. 2003. The quality of health care delivered to adults in the United States. *New England Journal of Medicine* 348(26):2635–2645.

Miller, D., L. Malley, and E. Owens. 2007. *Comparative indicators of education in the United States and other G-8 countries: 2006. (NCES 2007–006), US department of education.* Washington, DC: National Center for Educational Statistics

Napolitano, J. 2008. Executive order 2008–07: Reducing the escalation of health care costs for Arizonans. *Governor's Executive Orders/Proclamations* 14(5).

National Opinion Research Center. 2008. *AHRQ national resource center for health information technology.* http://www.norc.org/projects/ahrq+national+resource+center+for+health+information+technology.htm (accessed August 18, 2008).

Nielsen, J. 2005. *Usability: Empiricism or ideology?* http://www.useit.com/alertbox/20050627.html (accessed July 9, 2008).

Norman, C. D., and H. A. Skinner. 2006a. eHEALS: The eHealth literacy scale. *Journal of Medical Internet Research* 8(4):e27.

Norman, C. D., and H. A. Skinner. 2006b. eHealth literacy: Essential skills for consumer health in a networked world. *Journal of Medical Internet Research* 8(2):e9.

Oh, H., C. Rizo, M. Enkin, and A. Jadad. 2005. What is eHealth (3): A systematic review of published definitions. *Journal of Medical Internet Research* 7(1):e1.

Partnership for Solutions. 2004. *Chronic conditions: Making the case for ongoing care.* www.partnershipforsolutions.org/DMS/files/chronicbook2004.pdf. (accessed June 18, 2008).

PC Magazine. 2008. *Encyclopedia.* http://www.pcmag.com/encyclopedia_term/0,2542,t=RSS&i=50680,00.asp (accessed August 14, 2008).

Ratzan, S., and R. Parker. 2000. Introduction. In *National Library of Medicine current bibliographies in medicine: Health literacy*. NLM Pub. No. CBM 2000-1 ed., edited by C. Selden, M. Zorn, S. Ratzan, and R. Parker. Bethesda, MD: National Institutes of Health, U.S. Department of Health and Human Services.

Raymond, B., and C. Dold. 2002. *Clinical information systems: Achieving the vision.* Oakland, CA: Kaiser Permanente Institute for Health Policy.

Rodgers, A. 2008. *Strategies for raising health literacy in Arizona Medicaid members: New approaches for state Medicaid and "health knowledge builders."* Powerpoint presentation at the Institute of Medicine workshop on health literacy, eHealth, and communication: Putting the consumer first. Washington, DC, March 17.

Rubenson, K., R. Desjardins, and E. Yoon. 2007. *Adult learning in canada: A comparative persepective: Results from the adult literacy and life skills survey.* Ottowa, ON: Statistics Canada.

SearchMobileComputing.com. 2008. *Searchmobilecomputing.Com definitions.* http://searchmobilecomputing.techtarget.com/sDefinition/0,,sid40_gci838865,00.html (accessed August 14, 2008).

Seymour-Rolls, K., and I. Hughes. 2000. *Participatory action research: Getting the job done.* http://www2.fhs.usyd.edu.au/arow/arer/004.htm (accessed August 14, 2008).

Shea, K., A. Shih, and K. Davis. 2007. *Health care opinion leaders' views on the quality and safety of health care in the United States.* New York: The Commonwealth Fund

Shoen, C., S. How, I. Weinbaum, J. Craig Jr., and K. Davis. 2006. *Public views on shaping the future of the US health system.* New York: The Commonwealth Fund.

Skinner, H. A., S. Biscope, and B. Poland. 2003a. Quality of internet access: Barrier behind internet use statistics. *Social Science & Medicine* 57(5):875–880.

Skinner, H. A., S. Biscope, B. Poland, and E. Goldberg. 2003b. How adolescents use technology for health information: Implications for practitioners. *Journal of Medical Internet Research* 5(4):e32.

Solomon, C. 2008. *Using technology to improve migrant health care delivery.* Powerpoint presentation at the Institute of Medicine workshop on health literacy, eHealth, and communication: Putting the consumer first. Washington, DC, March 17.

Stamm, K., and R. Dube. 1994. The relationship of attitudinal components to trust in media. *Communication Research* 21(1):105–123.

Statistics Canada. 2005. *Building on our competencies: Canadian results of the international adult literacy and skills survey, 2003.* Ottawa, ON: Human Resources and Skills Development Canada and Statistics Canada.

Sussex Learning Network. 2006. *Glossary.* http://www.sussexlearningnetwork.org.uk/glossary/B (accessed August 14, 2008).

Techweb. 2008. *Techencyclopaedia: Streaming video.* http://www.techweb.com/encyclopedia/defineterm.jhtml?term=STREAMINGVIDEO (accessed August 14, 2008).

U.S. Bureau of the Census. 2000. *Projections of the total resident population by 5-year age groups and sex with special age categories: Middle series, 1999 to 2100. (np–t3)*. http://www.census.gov/population/www/projections/natsum-T3.html (accessed June 18, 2008).

Walker, J., E. Pan, D. Johnston, J. Adler-Milstein, D. Bates, and B. Middleton. 2005. The value of health care information exchange and interoperability. *Health Affairs (Millwood)* 19 Jan:10–18.

White, K., T. Williams, and B. Greenberg. 1961. The ecology of medical care. *New England Journal of Medicine* 265:885–892.

Wu, S., and A. Green. 2000. *Projection of chronic illness prevalence and cost inflation*. Santa Monica, CA: RAND Corporation.

Appendix A

Glossary of Terms

Bar Code Medication Administration (BCMA). "A point-of-care software solution that addresses the serious issue of inpatient medication errors by electronically validating and documenting medications for inpatients. It ensures that the patient receives the correct medication in the correct dose, at the correct time, and visually alerts staff when the proper parameters are not met" (http://www.innovations.va.gov/innovations/page.cfm?pg=13). Accessed July 5, 2008.

Blog. "A blog is a website where entries are made in journal style and displayed in a reverse chronological order. Blogs often provide commentary or news on a particular subject, such as food, politics, or local news; some function as more personal online diaries" (http://www.sussexlearningnetwork.org.uk/glossary/B). Accessed August 9, 2008.

eHealth. "Involves simplifying and handling processes relating to information, communication and transactions within and between health care institutions and professionals by utilizing information and telecommunications technologies" (www.interimreport.telekom.de/site0106/en/co/glossar/index.php).

Electronic Health Record (EHR). An EHR system includes "(1) longitudinal collection of electronic health information for and about persons, where health information is defined as information pertaining to the health of an individual or health care provided to an individual; (2) immediate electronic access to person- and population-level information by authorized, and only authorized, users; (3) provision of knowledge and decision-support that enhance the quality, safety, and efficiency of patient care; and (4) support of efficient processes for health care delivery. Critical building blocks of an EHR system are the electronic health records (EHR) maintained by providers (e.g., hospitals, nursing homes, ambulatory settings) and by individuals (also called personal health records)" (IOM, 2003).

Health literacy. "The degree to which individuals have the capacity to obtain, process, and understand basic health information and services needed to make appropriate health decisions" (Ratzan, S. C., and R. M. Parker. 2000. Introduction. In *National Library of Medicine Current Bibliographies in Medicine: Health Literacy*. NLM Pub. No. CBM 2000-1. C. R. Selden, M. Zorn, S. C. Ratzan, and R. M. Parker, Editors. Bethesda, MD: National Institutes of Health, U.S. Department of Health and Human Services).

Healthwise. "A nonprofit organization with a mission to help people make better health decisions. Nearly 100 million times a year, people turn to Healthwise information to learn how to do more for themselves, ask for the care they need, and say 'no' to the care they don't need. Healthwise partners with health plans, hospitals, disease management companies, and health Web sites to provide up-to-date, evidence-based information to the people they serve. To learn more about the Healthwise Information Therapy (Ix®) Solution, visit www.healthwise.org or call 1.800.706.9646" (http://hwinfo.healthwise.org/docs/DOCUMENT/9166.pdf). Accessed May 6, 2008.

HL7. "Health Level Seven is one of several American National Standards Institute (ANSI)-accredited Standards Developing Organizations (SDOs) operating in the healthcare arena. Health Level Seven's domain is clinical and administrative data" (http://www.hl7.org/). Accessed July 11, 2008.

Medical home. "A medical home is not just a building, house, or hospital, but a team approach to providing health care. A Medical Home originates in a primary health care setting that is family-centered and compassionate. A partnership develops between the family and the primary health care practitioner. Together they access all medical and non-medical services needed by the child and family to achieve maximum potential. The Medical Home maintains a centralized, comprehensive record of all health related services to promote continuity of care" (http://www.cdphe.state.co.us/ps/genetics/glossary.html#M). Accessed June 26, 2008.

MedLine Plus. A website network database of health information provided by the National Library of Medicine and the National Institutes of Health for use by consumers and health care providers.

Participatory Action Research (PAR). "A method of research where creating a positive social change is the predominant driving force" (http://www2.fhs.usyd.edu.au/arow/arer/004.htm). Accessed July 1, 2008.

PDA. A personal digital assistant is "a handheld device that combines computing, telephone/fax, Internet, and networking features. A typical PDA can function as a cellular phone, fax sender, Web browser, and personal organizer" (http://www.webopedia.com/TERM/P/PDA.html). Accessed August 11, 2008.

Personal Health Record (PHR). "An electronic Personal Health Record (ePHR) is a universally accessible, layperson comprehensible, lifelong tool for managing relevant health information, promoting health maintenance, and assisting with chronic disease management via an interactive, common data set of electronic health information and e-health tools. The ePHR is owned, managed, and shared by the individual or his or her legal proxy(s) and must be secure to protect the privacy and confidentiality of the health information it contains. It is not a legal record unless so defined and is subject to various legal limitations" (Healthcare Information and Management Systems Society. http://www.himss.org/asp/topics_phr.asp). Accessed August 11, 2008.

PODcast. "An audio broadcast that has been converted to an MP3 file or other audio file format for playback in a digital music player. Although many podcasts are played in a regular computer, the original idea was to listen on a portable device; hence, the 'pod' name from 'iPod.' Although podcasts are mostly verbal, they may contain music, images, and video" (http://www.pcmag.com/encyclopedia_term/0,2542,t=podcast&i=49433,00.asp). Accessed August 12, 2008.

Prevention Research Centers. "A network of academic researchers, public health agencies, and community members that conducts applied research in disease prevention and control" (http://www.cdc.gov/prc/). Accessed July 1, 2008.

RSS (Really Simple Syndication) Feed. "A syndication format that was developed by Netscape in 1999 and became very popular for aggregating updates to blogs and the news sites. RSS has also stood for "Rich Site Summary" (http://www.pcmag.com/encyclopedia_term/0,2542,t=RSS&i=50680,00.asp). Accessed August 11, 2008.

SOAP. The initials, SOAP, stand for subjective, objective, assessment plan. The SOAP format is used to document observations and care provided.

SSL. Secure sockets layer which is a technology used to protect websites.

Streaming Video. "A one-way video transmission over a data network. It is widely used on the Web as well as company networks to play video clips and video broadcasts" (http://www.techweb.com/encyclopedia/defineterm.jhtml?term=STREAMINGVIDEO). Accessed August 11, 2008.

Voucher sites. A voucher is an agreement between a provider and the voucher program (usually a migrant health grantee), to reimburse a provider, who is usually in a distant location, for health services provided to the migrant worker. Voucher sites are local providers who are contracted with on a per visit basis.

Web 1.0. Web 1.0 is "a general reference to the World Wide Web during its first few years of operation. The term is mostly used to contrast the earlier days of the Web before blogs, wikis, social networking sites and Web-based applications became commonplace" (http://dictionary.zdnet.com/definition/Web+1.0.html). Accessed November 3, 2008.

Web 2.0. "A term often applied to a perceived ongoing transition of the World Wide Web from a collection of websites to a full-fledged computing platform serving web applications to end users. It refers to a supposed second-generation of Internet-based services—such as social networking sites, wikis, communication tools, and folksonomies—that emphasize online collaboration and sharing among users" (http://www.2020systems.com/internet-ad-glossary-r-z.html). Accessed June 29, 2008.

Web portal. "A web portal is a term, often used interchangeably with gateway, for a World Wide Web site whose purpose is to be a major starting point for users when they connect to the Web" (http://www.mariosalexandrou.com/definition/web-portal.asp). Accessed August 11, 2008.

Wi-Fi. "Wi-Fi (short for 'wireless fidelity') is a term for certain types of wireless local area network (WLAN) that use specifications in the 802.11 family. The term Wi-Fi was created by an organization called the Wi-Fi Alliance, which oversees tests that certify product interoperability. A product that passes the alliance tests is given the label 'Wi-Fi certified' (a registered trademark)" (http://searchmobilecomputing.techtarget.com/sDefinition/0,,sid40_gci838865,00.html). Accessed August 11, 2008.

Wiki. "A wiki is a website that allows multiple users to create, modify, and organize web page content in a collaborative manner" (http://www.govst.edu/elearning/default.aspx?id=12984). Accessed August 9, 2008.

Wireframe. "A wireframe is a visualization tool for presenting proposed functions, structure and content of a Web page or Web site. A wireframe separates the graphic elements of a Web site from the functional elements in such a way that Web teams can easily explain how users will interact with the Web site. A typical wireframe includes (1) key page elements and their location, such as header, footer, navigation, content objects, branding elements, (2) grouping of elements, such as side bars, navigation bars, content areas, (3) labeling, page title, navigation links, headings to content objects, and (4) place holders, content text and images." (http://isp.webopedia.com/TERM/W/wireframe.html). Accessed July 9, 2008.

Appendix B

Workshop Agenda

Roundtable on Health Literacy
Institute of Medicine
Board on Population Health and Public Health Practice

Monday, March 17, 2008

Workshop on Health Literacy, eHealth, and Communication:
Putting the Consumer First

National Academies Building
2101 Constitution Avenue, NW
Washington, DC 20001

GOAL: To obtain information on the current status, barriers, and steps to be taken to facilitate eHealth strategies that incorporate needs of populations with low health literacy and language barriers.

OBJECTIVES: To organize presentations to address the following questions:
1. What is the current status of communication technology, particularly electronic health records systems?
2. What are the challenges of communication technology use for populations with low health literacy?
3. What are strategies for increasing the benefit of these technologies for populations with low health literacy?

MONDAY, MARCH 17, 2008

9:00-12:00 WORKSHOP SESSIONS—Lecture Room

9:00-9:15 Welcome and Overview
  George Isham
  Roundtable Chair

9:15-10:15	***Panel: Overview of the Issues***

9:15-9:35	Overview of eHealth. Presentation will address:
	1. What is eHealth
	2. What is the value of eHealth
	3. Definitions and status of
	   a. Internet use for health
	   b. Personal Health Records
	   c. Electronic clinical use (e.g., monitoring)
	Janet M. Marchibroda
	eHealth Initiative and eHealth Foundation

9:35-9:55	Skills Essential for eHealth 1. What is eHealth literacy? 2. What fundamental skills are needed to benefit from eHealth? **Cameron D. Norman** *University of Toronto*
9:55-10:15	Communication Inequalities and eHealth—challenges for populations with low health literacy and limited English proficiency **Anthony Rodgers** *Arizona Health Care Cost Containment System*
10:15-10:30	**BREAK**
10:30-11:00	Discussion
11:00-12:00	***Panel: Outcomes and Challenges—Some Examples***

Each panelist will discuss the project in which they are engaged, describing both outcomes achieved and the challenges encountered in addressing low health literacy or language barriers to the use of eHealth approaches.

11:00-11:20	Internet Approaches for eHealth in Low Literacy/LEP populations **Rita Kukafka** *Columbia University*

11:20-11:40	My Health*e*Vet ***Kim Nazi*** *Veterans Health Administration*	
11:40-12:00	Discussion	
12:00-1:00	**LUNCH**	
1:00-2:50	*Panel: Outcomes and Challenges—Some Examples (continued)*	

Each panelist will discuss the project in which they are engaged, describing both outcomes achieved and the challenges encountered.

1:00-1:20	MiVia ***Cynthia Solomon*** Medical Management Resources	
1:20-2:00	PeaceHealth ***Dawn Gauthier*** PeaceHealth	
2:00-2:20	Observations from the Exam Room: Patient-Centered HIT Implementation in Diverse Practice Settings. ***Joshua Seidman*** *Center for Information Therapy*	
2:20-2:50	Discussion	
2:50-3:15	**BREAK**	
3:15-3:35	A Guide for Developing and Purchasing Successful HIT ***Cindy Brach*** Agency for Healthcare Research and Quality	
3:35-4:00	Discussion	
4:00-4:30	Strategies for Integration ***Linda Harris*** ***Charles P. Friedman*** Department of Health and Human Services	
4:30-5:00	Discussion	

Appendix C

Workshop Speaker Biosketches

Cindy Brach, M.P.P., is a senior health policy researcher at the Agency for Healthcare Research and Quality (AHRQ). She is AHRQ's lead on cultural competence and sits on a number of cultural competence advisory groups. In addition to her own cultural competence research, she has overseen the development of guides to assist health plans in implementing culturally and linguistically appropriate services and a research agenda for cultural competence in health care. Currently, Ms. Brach is spearheading AHRQ's health literacy activities, coordinating AHRQ's work in developing measures and improving the evidence base, and integrating health literacy activities throughout AHRQ's portfolios.

Charles P. Friedman, Ph.D., is deputy national coordinator for Health Information Technology in the Office of the Secretary for Health and Human Services. In this capacity, he serves as the chief operating officer of the Office of the National Coordinator (ONC), working to build collaborations in the public and private sectors, and maintain cohesion across the programs that ONC undertakes. In addition, Dr. Friedman is ONC's lead for planning and communication activities, as well as the Office's initiatives relating to clinical decision support. He also lends his informatics expertise as needed to support activities of the Office.

Prior to joining the ONC, Dr. Friedman was institute associate director for Research Informatics and Information Technology at the National Heart, Lung, and Blood Institute of the National Institutes of Health. From 1996 to 2003, Dr. Friedman was professor and associate vice chancellor for biomedical informatics at the University of Pittsburgh. He established a well-funded program of informatics research and directed the enterprise-wide effort to develop and deploy integrated advanced information resources across the health sciences center. Dr. Friedman's research has focused on how to build information and knowledge resources that make clinicians, biomedical researchers, and health professional students better at what they do—and how to study the effects of these resources. He has also studied and written about how institutions can organize to make optimal use of their information and knowledge resources.

Dr. Friedman has authored or co-authored over 150 articles in scientific journals. He is the author of a well-known textbook on evaluation methods for biomedical informatics. He is a past president of the American College of Medical Informatics and was the 2005 chair of the Annual Symposium of the American Medical Informatics Association. He currently serves as associate editor of the *Journal of the American Medical Informatics Association*.

Dawn Gauthier, M.I.S., is a Web usability designer at PeaceHealth, a nonprofit six-hospital system based in Bellevue, Washington. From 2002 to 2006 she led the design and development of the Web-based *Shared Care Plan* personal health record (PHR), widely recognized for trailblazing many innovative and patient-centered PHR concepts. She also participated in an AHRQ-funded study on how patient-owned PHRs could be used to help maintain accurate medication lists across a community. More recently she has led the introduction of user-centered design and user experience to PeaceHealth's Web application development lifecycle. Ms. Gauthier holds a Master of Information Science degree, specializing in human-computer interaction, user-oriented information architecture, and interactive design, from Indiana University in Bloomington, Indiana. She currently resides in Bellingham, Washington, with her husband and passionately advocates for user-centered design in all health care processes, with an emphasis on patient needs and their privacy.

Linda Harris, Ph.D., leads the Health Communication and ehealth Team in the U.S. Department of Health and Human Services, Office of Disease Prevention and Health Promotion (ODPHP). In this role she supervises the management of the National Health Information Center, a congressionally mandated source of health information for the public (healthfinder.gov). Prior to her arrival at ODPHP, Dr. Harris was a senior health communication scientist at the National Cancer Institute, Division of Cancer Control and Population Sciences where she managed health communication technology research projects, including health systems research in collaboration with the VA. She has over 20 years of experience managing information technology/communication research and development projects in public health and in the private health care sector. She has extensive experience architecting, designing, developing, and evaluating information systems for consumers and health professionals. She is the editor of *Health and the New Media: Technologies Transforming Personal and Public Health*. Her Ph.D. is in communication from the University of Massachusetts.

Rita Kukafka, Dr.P.H., M.A., is jointly appointed with the Department of Biomedical Informatics and the Mailman School of Pubic Health (Sociomedical Sciences). She holds a doctorate degree from the School of Public Health at Columbia University and two master's degrees, one in health education, and the second in biomedical informatics from Columbia University, where she also completed a National Library of Medicine awarded postdoctoral fellowship in medical informatics.

Dr. Kukafka maintains an active, funded program of research and publication in public health informatics while being engaged in major leadership roles in the field. Her research is at the crossroads of biomedical informatics and public health including computer interventions for chronic disease self-management, health promotion and informed decision-making, patient focused electronic health records and personal health records, tailoring health communication, and interactive computer graphics for communicating health risk probabilities to patients. Another area of her research focuses on how theory from the behavioral sciences can be applied to advance our understanding and to improve our capacity to implement information technology systems into health care organizations. She is a member of the American Medical Informatics Association Board of Directors and she is a past chair of that organization's Working Group on Consumer Health Informatics. She is on the editorial board of the *Journal of Biomedical Informatics*, and serves on the editorial boards for several other biomedical informatics publications. Dr. Kukafka has authored several key articles and books, and book chapters in the fields of public health informatics and consumer health informatics.

Dr. Kukafka is an experienced mentor; notably in the area of public health informatics where she spearheaded the formation of the public health informatics program at the Department of Biomedical Informatics, Columbia University, one of four programs in the country, to build this specialization with training support from the Robert Wood Foundation and National Library of Medicine.

Janet M. Marchibroda, M.B.A., is the chief executive officer of the eHealth Initiative and its Foundation, both Washington, DC-based independent, national nonprofit organizations whose missions are to improve the quality, safety and efficiency of health care through information and information technology.

The eHealth Initiative is a multi-stakeholder member organization—representing clinicians, employers, health plans, health care IT suppliers, hospitals and other health care providers, consumer groups, pharmaceutical and medical device manufacturers, public health organizations, standards bodies, and academic institutions—that develops consensus among multiple and diverse stakeholders on strategies that will drive better health care for patients through the use of information technology. Through the eHealth Initiative Foundation, the organization provides financial and technical support to state, regional, and community-based multi-stakeholder collaboratives across the nation who are mobilizing health information electronically to support patient care.

Ms. Marchibroda previously served as the executive director of Connecting for Health—a public–private sector initiative funded and led by the Markle Foundation and supported by the Robert Wood Johnson Foundation—which is designed to catalyze actions on a national basis to drive electronic connectivity and create an interconnected, electronic health information infrastructure. In addition, she was recognized in 2005 as one of the Top 25 Women in Healthcare by Modern Healthcare magazine and in 2006 for the Federal Computer Week Top 100 Award.

Prior to the eHealth Initiative, Ms. Marchibroda cofounded and served as chief operating officer for two health care information organizations, one which focuses on providing patient safety and compliance information to physicians and the other—a Bertelsmann AG subsidiary—which focuses on providing electronic publishing services to the payer community to support member information needs. She also served as the interim chief operating officer for the National Coalition for Cancer Survivorship.

Ms. Marchibroda also served as the chief operating officer of the National Committee for Quality Assurance, an organization devoted to evaluating and improving the quality of health care for Americans—where she was responsible for accreditation of health care organizations, education programs, the national HEDIS database, electronic information products, strategic planning, human resources, finance, and administration. She holds a B.S. in commerce from the University of Virginia and an M.B.A. with a concentration in organization development from George Washington University.

Kim Nazi, F.A.C.H.E., is a management analyst for the Department of Veterans Affairs (VA), working in the Veterans/Consumer Health Informatics Office of the Veterans Health Administration (VHA). She is a Board-Certified Healthcare Executive and a fellow in the American College of Healthcare Executives. She holds a master's degree in strategic communication from Seton Hall University, New Jersey and is currently a doctoral student in the joint sociology/communication program at the University of Albany. Ms. Nazi's research interests include technology and personal health records, health communication, and behavioral interventions. Prior to taking on her current role in July 2006, she served as the director of eHealth for the VA Healthcare Network Upstate New York, focusing on the use of technology to improve and expand the delivery of health care services. Ms. Nazi is a graduate of the VA's Executive Career Field Candidate program and a member of the American Health Information Community Consumer Empowerment Workgroup.

Cameron D. Norman, Ph.D., is an assistant professor in the Department of Public Health Sciences at the University of Toronto, director of evaluation with the Peter A. Silverman Global eHealth Program, and the principal investigator of Youth Voices Research, the youth engagement unit of the Centre for Health Promotion. The focus of his research is on understanding how people work together to solve health problems and how information technologies can aid learning and collaboration across time, physical space, and culture to improve health and well-being. His current research is seeking to understand how youth and young adults are engaged in health promotion through virtual communities; exploring what skills are necessary to fully participate in health decisions using information technology (eHealth); and how social networks connect ideas together to translate knowledge into improved health practices with professionals and consumers alike. Dr. Norman has published and presented widely on the concept of *eHealth literacy*, which he developed (with Harvey Skinner at York University) as a means of framing the essential skills necessary to fully engage with electronic health tools. His eHealth Literacy Scale is currently in use in nine countries and has been translated into five languages and applied to both consumer and health professional populations.

Dr. Norman holds a Ph.D. in public health from the University of Toronto and completed a post-doctoral fellowship in systems thinking and complexity science jointly at the University of British Columbia and the Centre for Global eHealth Innovation in Toronto. He lives in Toronto.

Anthony "Tony" Rodgers has over 25 years of health care executive management experience in both hospital systems and health plans. He currently holds the position of director of the Arizona Medicaid Program, known as the Arizona Health Care Cost Containment System.

As Director, Mr. Rodgers reports to the Governor and is responsible for providing health coverage for one million Arizonans. The agency administers multiple sources of funding and provides oversight and compliance to health care providers that focus on quality of care and fiscal accountability.

Mr. Rodgers currently holds visiting professor appointments at Arizona State University, at the W.P Carey School of Business, and at University of California–Los Angeles, School of Public Health.

Joshua Seidman, Ph.D., M.H.S., has been on a quest to improve health care quality for 17 years—first by influencing health plans and provider behavior, then shifting to a grassroots approach by activating consumers. In October 2001, Dr. Seidman saw the fusion of his two strategies to improve health care quality in information therapy. Information therapy (Ix) is the timely prescription and availability of evidence-based health information to meet individuals' specific needs and support sound decision making.

Dr. Seidman leads the independent, not-for-profit IxCenter and provides key leadership and direction, applying his extensive experience in strategic planning, product development, research, and education.

Before launching the IxCenter, Dr. Seidman served as senior editor and director of quality initiatives for the Advisory Board Company's Consumer Health Initiative. In that capacity, he played a leading role in strategic planning and product development and provided leadership in the development of quality-of-care information for consumers.

Dr. Seidman has worked for the National Committee for Quality Assurance as the director of measure development, overseeing analytical projects related to health-plan-performance measure testing and development for HEDIS®. He has also worked at the Advisory Board Company as a consultant and at the American College of Cardiology as assistant director of Private Sector Relations, conducting extensive research and analysis in managed care, quality-of-care issues, and other aspects of the health care industry. In addition, Dr. Seidman has published several book chapters and articles in peer-reviewed journals on eHealth and quality-of-care-related issues.

Dr. Seidman holds a Ph.D. in health services research and a master of health science degree in health policy and management, both from the Johns Hopkins School of Public Health. His doctoral research involved the development of a tool to evaluate the quality of health information on the Internet and an assessment of what website characteristics influenced health information quality. He earned a bachelor of arts in political science from Brown University.

Due to his unique dissertation research and expertise, he has served as a consultant to independent oversight groups and government agencies in the assessment of electronic consumer health information, and has served as a peer reviewer for various scientific journals including *The*

Journal of Medical Internet Research. He also authored the California Health-Care Foundation Issue Brief, "Lost in Translation: Consumer Health Information in an Interoperable World," which examines what could be done to better integrate consumer health information standards into PHRs and the national health information network framework.

For 5 years, Dr. Seidman volunteered as president of the board of directors for Micah House, a transitional house in Washington, DC, for homeless women recovering from substance abuse. Seidman uses distance running as his own therapy of sorts, and has completed 27 marathons.

Cynthia Solomon is CEO of Access Strategies Inc, a health care consulting firm located in Sonoma, California. Her company specializes in research, development and implementation of special projects which focus on systems of care for at-risk populations including the indigent, chronically ill and uninsured. She has over 25 years experience as a health systems consultant in the private and public health sectors. Ms. Solomon is a cofounder of MiVia, an electronic personal health record for migrant and seasonal workers developed for a nonprofit coalition of health and service providers serving agricultural workers. In October 2005, MiVia was highlighted in the Presidential Commission Report on Systemic Interoperability, submitted to Congress (www.endingthedocumentgame.gov). MiVia is currently being implemented in California, Oregon, and two rural migrant health networks in New York.

Ms. Solomon's company launched the FollowMe™ PHR in 2000. The FollowMe platform has been recognized as a pioneer in the field of PHRs and has been featured in several national publications including *The Economist*, *Washington Post*, *Wall Street Journal*, *L.A. Times*, *Medical Ethics*, and *For the Record*. She is a member of the Markle Foundation *Connecting for Health* Workgroup and participated in developing the recommendations and standards for interoperability between electronic health records (EHRs) and PHRs which was submitted to the Office of the National Coordinator for Health Information Technology (HHS) in July 2004. Ms. Solomon has presented testimony on PHR technology to the NCVHS NHII workgroup in April 2005. She has also presented testimony to the Consumer Empowerment Workgroup–American Health Information Community on the role of Government in PHR technology.

As the mother of a child diagnosed with hydrocephalus she is an experienced and committed health advocate and cofounder of the Hydrocephalus Association, a national support and advocacy organization for families and individuals living with hydrocephalus. Her son Alex has had multiple procedures and hospitalizations and it was her frustration with trying to manage and coordinate his complex medical information that led her to developing a Web-based PHR in 1999.